Raves from Sensa Users

"All I can say is—WOW! I don't know how this stuff works or why this stuff works but it DOES work (much to my amazement!). I have tried many 'miracle' products in the past. Pills to raise energy, to make you feel full, to burn off that fat even while you sleep. None of them helped even though I was going to the gym 2 to 3 times a week and I'm an avid swimmer. I didn't think it would work. I didn't expect it to work. I was sure I was throwing my money away but you all know what desperation will make you do—try anything! And it worked! As simple as that—it worked! The product is so remarkable."

R.

"This is the best thing I've ever done weight-loss wise. Wish it had been around 30 years ago when I was younger and was running around after kids."

S.

"I HAVE LOST 9½ LBS in just 4 weeks. This is a miracle. I eat what I enjoy, never feel deprived, not jittery. Just wonderful I am gaining my confidence back. My husband tells me I am looking great and walking taller!!! Thank you so much for changing my life!!!!!!!"

J. F.

"For post menopausal women, losing weight becomes even more challenging. Increasing exercise daily and diets no longer helped. Sensa has been a revelation! The science behind Dr. Hirsch's treatment made perfect sense, but the results are amazing. It has been three weeks, and I have lost 6lbs. with ease and never a sense of hunger or deprivation. I was so impressed with the product's performance; I shared this with my endocrinologist who will be suggesting Sensa to his patients with weight loss difficulties. The safety and efficacy make this the best weight management tool I have ever encountered."

A. R.

"I am overjoyed; I can't believe it and I feel wonderful, euphoric, satisfied, pleasant, un-victimized by cravings and totally normal . . . for the first time in my life. I LOVE IT! It is just heavenly and I thank the wonderful doctor profusely for this amazing product."

D.

"I can't believe the results I have gotten with Sensa and it has been so easy! I am just about to start month 3 and I have already lost about 8 lbs. Everyone is noticing the change already. My daughter-in-law and her friend are going to start using it too. This product has been lifesaving for me"

S. N.

"I am 57 years old. I am so thrilled with Sensa. I have been using it for almost 3 months, and I have lost 16 pounds. I have never before been able to lose weight so fast and easily. From the beginning, it made such a difference. I wasn't hungry all of the time, and was satisfied with much smaller portions. I have never felt that I am dieting or depriving myself. My husband went on the program with me, and has experienced the same success. I am so happy for him, because he needed to lose the weight for health reasons, to lower his blood pressure. Thanks to you Sensa. I can't wait to complete the six month program and be at least 30 pounds lighter."

J. H.

"I can honestly say that after just a day or two of using Sensa, I noticed I was not craving food as often. I am only a week into my second month, but my eating pattern has changed considerably—I eat the same foods I always have, but I don't eat as often simply because I don't have a desire to. It is truly amazing! I have lost six pounds."

L. C.

"Well, it's been 9 days since I started with Sensa and I really can't believe the results so far. I've lost 4.5 pounds and I've really changed nothing about my diet other than sprinkling Sensa and drinking more water! I was so skeptical at first, I mean really skeptical to the point where I almost cancelled my order. But I'm glad that I didn't, I'm really losing weight."

C.

"It's been 6 weeks and I've lost 13 pounds so far. It's so easy. I don't have to say NO when invited out. I can still go out to dinner. No special food. LOVE IT!"

J. V.

"I am having great success with your product. I lost 20 lbs in 2 months. I am very happy with the results so far."

M. H.

"I have recently just started using Sensa. It really does curb your appetite. I have already lost 5 lbs. I would recommend this to anyone."

T. H.

"I have actually lost 8 lbs. I can't believe it. I ate really everything I wanted. I even had potato chips and a dish of ice cream for snack this week! This is so easy! I can do this! I'm a believer now! Thanks Sensa and Dr. Hirsch. I'll keep you posted!"

J. F.

"I have lost 45 lbs to date. Most people I tell about Sensa just can't believe that it helps to control hunger. Each week when I visit with friends I am able to report that I lost 3 lbs again in the past week. This has been an easy way to help control hunger and lose weight. Those that have a view that is can't be true, just need to believe and give it a try."

C. M.

"I am on my fourth month with Sensa. I love it. My nickname at work is Sprinkles. Whenever anyone sees me eat they see me sprinkle my Sensa on all my food. I have lost 15 lbs so far. I am so excited I will probably stay on Sensa for the rest of my life. It is the best way to lose weight. Sensa has become a way of life for me. It is so easy and if you give it a chance it will pay you back by working for you."

P. S.

"Lost 30 lbs in 4 months!"

J. C.

"I have gained weight throughout the years due to steroids and exercise for me is a little bit difficult at times. I think as I get older it's harder to lose weight. However with Sensa I lost 18 pounds in three months and look and feel great. I am finally feeling me again!!! Thank you!!!"

L. F.

"I have been on Sensa for a month now. I sprinkle it on everything. I have not really changed what I eat. But I am more aware of what I eat. I have lost 6 lbs. I do not exercise as of yet and I do drink on weekends. I have no side affects and did not believe it would work but it has. It's great! I feel much better about myself too. My husband has even noticed the change in my weight and attitude. Thanks Sensa!!!!!"

S. L.

"My neighbor told me about Sensa and I thought it sounded silly, but after 2 months I am sold!! On my last Dr. visit I had lost 12 pounds and I am delighted with Sensa results. I too, was skeptical but would recommend it!!!"

L. B.

"I have been on Sensa for 1 month & I lost 8 lbs. I just started my 2nd month & am looking forward to losing more weight. Thanks."

G. F.

"I saw Sensa on TV and immediately went to your website. THIS HAS TRANS-FORMED ME & MY BODY. I have been on Sensa now for 7 months, lost 18 pounds and lost several inches. Everyone at work has noticed the difference & I've been giving out the DVD so others can have the same success. Thank you for this great product!"

B. E.

"I can't believe this is happening to me. I have lost 10 pounds in 6 weeks! I tried the diet where food is delivered to you. Not only was it very expensive but I only lost 10 pounds in 9 months and I stuck to it 100%. What is so wonderful with SENSA is I'm never STARVING anymore. When I go out for a meal I only eat 1/3 of it because I'm full! Thanks Doc!"

N. T.

"This was truly unbelievable. I'll admit it did sound much too good to be true. I began the program and saw immediate results within the first week. I am two and half weeks into my second month and have achieved my goal of losing 14 pounds! I am at a very healthy BMI for the first time since having my babies. I know that Sensa was the difference. I feel great and I can't begin to tell everyone how wonderful it is to be satisfied from a meal without feeling the need to have more food. Again, the results are unbelievable but I am living proof to the reality of this amazing product. It works! Do your part and Sensa does the hard part for you. Many thanks."

B. M.

"I have lost 17 lbs. in less than 3 months."

W. B.

"I'm on week 11 and down 18 lbs."

J. C.

"I was a compulsive eater. Sensa makes me so much more aware of what I am eating and how much. I now eat less and I am not hungry between meals. I can go longer without picking at food. It might not be your miracle but it is mine."

P. S.

"I weighed in again this morning and lost another pound and a half! I'm 133! Unbelievable. I am a true believer in this product. My husband started the program as well once he saw my loss and has lost 13 pounds himself! We recently added to our life insurance policy and were both rated as "preferred" because we are so healthy. WE LOVE SENSA!!!!!!!"

B. M.

"I am convinced without doubt that Sensa has changed my life. Instead of aimlessly stuffing myself all day, I am now enjoying eating small portions that are filling and long satisfying. I spent a lifetime letting food control me and my emotions . . . no more . . . I am in charge now. I feel like I have been let out of prison. Sensa has enabled me to feel normal about food, for the first time in my life. I eat normal, feel full and stop. Wow! What a concept!

P. D.

"My fridge is no longer in charge of my life. Thank you Sensa. I dread scales. Hate having to do weigh-ins at the doctor's as well as at home. But now I am excited. I'm EXCITED to WEIGH myself and I even checked my calendar for my next doctor appointment because I can't wait until he sees how much weight I've lost. During my last appointment he was discussing surgery. Thank you. Thank you Sensa!"

R. E.

"I took a chance with Sensa. To my extreme delight it has worked far beyond what I ever imagined. I've said it before . . . this to me is not a diet . . . I'm far too happy and content. I'm now down 17 lbs. 10 ounces from my starting weight of 217. I haven't been below 200 for over 2 decades."

E. W.

"So here I am into my second month. It hasn't been hard. I was always too ashamed of my obesity to admit it. I hid behind it and wouldn't discuss it with anyone, let alone tell the whole world what I was doing.

So, where did all this strength come from? I'm not sure where, but I do know one thing . . . I like it and I'm not going to stop!"

S. S.

"I am down 5 pounds as of today. Sensa has taught me to really think about what I am eating."

S. P.

"I have been using Sensa for 7 weeks and almost down 8 pounds. I am down a pant size. I am 58 and in menopause so I am really happy."

B. B.

SENSA®

WEIGHT-LOSS
PROGRAM

[
The Accidental Discovery
That's Transforming the Way
People Lose Weight
]

- Eat all your favorite foods
- Clinically proven results
- No restrictive dieting

Alan Hirsch, M.D., F.A.C.P.

Hilton Publishing
Chicago, Illinois

© 2009 by Alan R. Hirsch, M.D.

Hilton Publishing Company
Chicago, IL

Direct all correspondence to:
Hilton Publishing Company
1630 45th Street, Suite 103
Munster, IN 46321
219–922–4868
www.hiltonpub.com

ISBN 978–0–9841447–1–6 (Paperback)
ISBN 978–0–9815381–8–1 (Hardcover)

Notice: The information in this book is true and complete to the best of the author's and publisher's knowledge. Always consult your physician before starting any weight-loss and exercise plan. This book is intended only as an informative reference and should not replace, countermand, or conflict with the advice given to readers by their physicians. The Sensa Weight-Loss System may not be effective if you have an impaired or diminished sense of smell or taste. The authors and publisher disclaim all liability in connection with the specific personal use of any and all information provided in this book. Some references to real people, events, establishments, organizations, or locales are intended only to provide a sense of authenticity and are used fictitiously. However, references to success stories are real and permission has been granted by the individuals profiled in Chapter 9. Individual weight loss results may vary. The results shared in the Sensa Success Stories are not typical.

Library of Congress Cataloging-in-Publication Data

Hirsch, Alan R.
    Sensa: the book / by Alan R. Hirsch.
        p. cm.
    ISBN 978–0–9841447–1–6 (Paperback)
    ISBN 978–0–9815381–8–1 (Hardcover)
    1. Weight Loss. 2. Hunger. 3. Taste. 4. Smell. I. Title.
    RM222.2.H565 2008   612.8—dc22

Printed and bound in the United States of America

This book is dedicated to the memory of my father, Milton Hirsch, whose lifetime struggle with obesity and its effects inspired me to devote my life to working in the areas of smell, taste, and ultimately their connection to weight loss.

Contents

CONTENTS

PART II
THE SENSA WEIGHT-LOSS PROGRAM

Foreword

I first met Dr. Hirsch in 1991 when I was a medical student at the University of Illinois, rotating in my neurology clerkship at Mercy Medical Center on the south side of Chicago. Dr. Hirsch was well known to the medical student community as being not only an empathic clinician, but also an outstanding teacher, who spent the time and energy to make sure students learned the essentials and basics of neurology.

Early on, Dr. Hirsch introduced me to a patient who had experienced severe head trauma after being thrown off his motorcycle. In his kind, gentle way, Dr. Hirsch explained that the man's brain damage included an unusual form of aphasia, or inability to speak. This isolation aphasia, means that the brain areas involved in hearing, repeating, and speaking were intact, but segregated from the rest of the brain. As a result, all the patient could do was repeat things, much like a human parrot. He repeated words and sounds but had no idea what they meant, nor could he follow commands. If a bell rang, he mimicked the noise that the bell made. Being unable to make any spontaneous speech on his own distressed him. He couldn't ask for anything or express a desire. When Dr. Hirsch examined this patient, it was the first time I had ever seen any doctor test a patient's sense of smell. He held a vial of vanilla up to the patient's nose and, incredibly, a wide smile came over the patient's face. This patient who had been in such a horrible, painful accident, with such marked, frustrating neurological deficits, was thrilled to know that his ability to smell was intact and that he could, in some way, express how he felt. From then on, I was intrigued by the relationships among the sense of smell, the brain, and human behavior.

During the next few years I worked with Dr. Hirsch to conduct studies of medications to improve patients' smell loss. At the Smell & Taste Treatment and Research Foundation in Chicago, I had previously assisted Dr. Hirsch in his early studies of using smells to help treat obesity.

We spent many long hours researching to see if odors could enhance learning. I was often strapped into a coffin-like tube as we explored how odors affected claustrophobia. When residents, medical students, and fellows encountered obstacles to our research, Dr. Hirsch frequently reminded us that "perfection is a journey, not a destination." His guidance helped propel me into the world of neurotherapeutics and ultimately to my position as an Associate Professor of Psychiatry at Harvard Medical School.

In *The Sensa Weight-Loss Program*, Dr. Hirsch cogently presents a remarkable and overlooked approach to weight loss. By using the body's senses of smell and taste, he has been able to develop an entire weight loss program that offers solid results. His instincts and research into the smell-taste-weight connection ultimately led to the groundbreaking discoveries outlined in this book. I have seen first hand the results of Dr. Hirsch's research in the long-term management of obesity accompanied by sustained weight loss. Dr. Hirsch's approach overcomes the negative aspects of weight loss including dieting and restrictions, and therefore helps people stay on the program. Dr. Hirsch's program also involves unconscious mechanisms to maximize the perception of "feeling full," or satiety. This approach has the potential of helping millions of people in the United States and billions of people worldwide who suffer from the indignities and adverse health effects of being overweight. I encourage all to read this book and try Dr. Hirsch's approach. You will be amazed and gratified by the results.

Darin Dougherty, M.D.
Director, Division of Neurotherapeutics
Department of Psychiatry, Massachusetts
General Hospital
Associate Professor of Psychiatry,
Harvard Medical School

Introduction

WELCOME TO A NEW WAY OF LOSING WEIGHT

For more than twenty-five years, my work has focused on the care and treatment of people with smell and taste disorders. Patients come to the Smell & Taste Treatment and Research Foundation in Chicago from all over the world looking for reasons, answers, and cures to their conditions.

Like many of us who "fall" into a particular profession, I had no intention of becoming a specialist in this area. After completing medical school and my internship, I did my residency in neurology—the study of the nervous system—where I learned how to diagnose, treat, and manage disorders such as Parkinson's disease, multiple schlerosis, Lou Gehrig's disease (aka Amyotrophic Lateral Sclerosis or ALS), migraines, epilepsy, and neck and back pain.

I discovered that many of my patients who were affected by these disabling and often very painful neurological disorders also suffered substantial depression and anxiety about their conditions.

Not only were patients themselves depressed, but their family members were equally devastated and depressed as a result of caring for and worrying about their parents, children, or spouses. Yet, the issues of psychological distress went unrecognized and ignored by the medical profession.

As I spent more and more time talking to these patients, I realized that treating just their diseases and disorders didn't address the entire patient or solve their related problems. I began to see that a more holistic approach—treating the whole patient, not just the primary neurological disorder—would benefit them to a far greater degree than simply addressing their primary neurological complaints. After completing four years of neurology residency, I studied for another four more years, completing a residency in psychiatry.

With my background and training in neurology, I performed full neurological examinations on all my psychiatric inpatients. I was shocked by what I found. Patients who were admitted for schizophrenia, bipolar illness, or manic-depressive disorder often had no sense of smell. Had I come upon the missing link for understanding psychiatric disease? Was this a potential biological marker of psychological disorders? Could an objective abnormality, not requiring patient's complaints, be used to help identify underlying mental disorders? I tested all of my patients and kept replicating my findings; that they could not smell. I spent all of my free time looking at the potential connection between olfactory ability and psychiatric disorders. What I ultimately discovered was that these patients couldn't smell due to the psychotropic medications they were taking including: neuroleptics, Thorazine, Haldol, and Lithium. This major side effect wasn't mentioned in the drug literature. I could have kicked myself for not realizing this sooner. By the time I discovered this, I was already so well immersed in the area of smell and taste. I just continued my studies.

Over the years, I began to see more patients with smell and taste disorders and fewer with general neurological and psychiatric problems. One of the many things I noticed was that when people lost their sense of smell, they became more anxious. This suggested a possible connection between smell loss and anxiety, or to the contrary, perhaps some sort of ambient relaxant in the air that we all smell, and when we lose our sense of smell, we can't detect it and thus we become anxious. My colleagues and I began doing studies on the effects of odors on anxiety. We discovered through group therapy sessions that people who lost their sense of smell became claustrophobic and couldn't bear to ride in elevators, so we began to explore how odors can affect spacial perception, or room size. Based on our clinical material, we began to explore how odors affected exercise strength, migraine headaches, claustrophobia, agoraphobia, learning behavior, sexual arousal, and weight loss. We even found that the ability to detect some odors could be used as a diagnostic tool for some diseases.

For instance, when we discovered that women with estrogen-positive breast carcinoma, a form of breast cancer, often had an impaired ability to smell, we worked on developing an olfactory test that could be used as an alternative to mammography or to help determine reoccurrence of the disease early on. This is an area we are continuing to explore.

We found that levels of depression, based on a test called the Beck Depression Inventory, correlated with the ability to smell specific artificial odors. As a result, we have been working for the last twenty years on a specific olfactory assay, or olfactory test, to help determine if patients who are depressed and on antidepressants need to have their antidepressant doses raised or lowered.

We extensively studied the effects of odors on hand-eye coordination, looking at the effects on sports activity such as bowling, riding a stationary bicycle, and even looking at free-throw rates in NBA players in the presence of different odors.

We performed multiple studies on the effects of unpleasant odors on aggression and anger, along with the potential use of more pleasant odors as a way of minimizing aggression and enhancing social ability.

We gave 18,631 patients a battery of psychological tests to determine personality type and correlated this with how much they liked or disliked certain foods and smells. Originally designed for use by psychiatrists to help diagnose different conditions, we found that anyone could use these tests in many areas. Employment agencies and trial attorneys have even utilized these studies to help determine employability and likelihood of conviction rate.

We learned that there is an entire invisible universe of smells, aromas, and odors waiting to be explored. Our sense of smell impacts everything we do—how we live, shop, eat, sleep, exercise, and relate to others around us. When we noted that patients who lost their senses of smell and taste after significant trauma gained weight, we followed our hunches and explored how the senses of smell and taste, and weight were connected to one another. This ultimately led to the discovery of a revolutionary, scientifically proven, and effective way to lose weight.

How To Use This Book

In the following pages, you'll learn how your senses of smell and taste are powerful tools that can be used to control your appetite and maintain a healthy weight. You'll read about other people who used this discovery to successfully lose weight. You'll see how this remarkable program delivers on its promise to the millions of people who want to lose weight.

Before jumping into the "how to" portion of the book, it is important to understand the epidemic of overeating, the role that smell and taste play in our lives, to discover a new way of looking at being overweight. It's OK to want to get started on the 3–step program right away, but I designed the first half of the book as a way to understand your body and to motivate you on your new journey. It's up to you to figure out your pace. No matter what chapter you start with, you will find a new approach to tackle the challenges of weight loss and breakthrough to a thinner you.

PART I

THE SCIENCE
BEHIND SENSA

Chapter 1

YOUR JOURNEY TO A NEW YOU

When you first saw this book, you were probably attracted to it by either the title or the words "weight loss" on the cover. You are probably one of the thousands of people today that are interested in losing a few pounds or a lot of weight. When you first picked the book up, you probably looked at the front, read some of the testimonials on the back, read the inside jacket and then you wanted to see how the first chapter started out. You were "testing the water" so to speak, to see if this book would be different from the hundreds of other weight loss books on the market today. Was I right?

Now let me give you the answer—what you are about to experience in this book is totally different from any other weight loss book that you have read or followed. This book approaches weight loss in a completely unique way, in a way that is the simplest, easiest, safest and most effective program ever developed. And the best part is that this program was completely discovered by accident.

The Accidental Discovery

When you look at the area of new product inventions, some of the greatest ones have been discovered by accident. In fact, there is an old saying that states that good inventions are often born out of need, but great ones are discovered by accident.

In 1928, an absent-minded biologist, Sir Alexander Fleming was researching a strain of bacteria called staphylococci. Upon returning from a holiday absence, he noticed that one of the glass culture dishes that he had left out had become contaminated with a fungus. Later, he noticed that the bacteria that he was researching were unable to grow outside of the boundaries of this fungus. Years after publishing his findings, scientists took note and the first commercial production of penicillin took place that changed the medical world forever.

In 1945 Percy Spencer was experimenting with a new vacuum tube for the company Raytheon. While doing his experimentation, he noticed that the candy bar in his pocket began to melt. He put two and two together and tried the same experiment using popcorn. When the popcorn began to pop, he realized that this accidental discovery could fill a need and hence, the first microwave oven was born.

In 1980, Pfizer, the large pharmaceutical company, started experimenting with a drug that evolved into a treatment for angina. The drug was eventually deemed a failure but researchers noticed a curious side effect—an erection in males suffering from erectile dysfunction. Needless to say, Pfizer noticed a huge market for this product and Viagra has since become the fastest growth drug product in history.

The Pleasure/Pain Principle

If you are still "testing the water" in deciding about this book, there are probably numerous other questions that you are asking yourself:

> "Will this be the answer—will this be the magic pill that I'm looking for?"
> "Will this book help me to get back to my ideal weight?"
> "How difficult is this program going to be?"
> "How much work is this going to take?"
> "How much am I going to have to deviate from my normal routine?"
> "How much pain am I going to have to endure?"

This last question probably hit home more than any of the others—"how much pain am I going to have to endure"?

The "Pleasure/Pain Principle" states that humans are driven by two basic principles; they seek pleasure and avoid pain. When the two drivers are in conflict, humans typically seek to avoid pain first. One of the areas that this principle aptly applies to is the area of dieting. In fact, just the word "dieting" conjures up all kinds of negative emotions and feelings of pain, including drastic deprivation and lifestyle changes. There is nothing pleasurable about the concept of dieting.

But what if you could achieve weight loss without the feeling of pain, without the feeling of deprivation, without the feeling of having your world turned upside down in the hope of losing a few pounds? What would you think about this? You would probably say, "That sounds too good to be true." And we have always been taught, that if something sounds too good to be true, then it probably is. But let's look at some of the inventions that we spoke about earlier. In 1928, would people have been skeptical if we had said that we invented something that would allow us to dramatically lower the incidence of infectious diseases, conduct open heart surgery and transplant human organs? The accidental discovery of penicillin accomplished this. In 1945, what would we have found out if we had taken a survey of the population and told them that instead of using a stove, we had a small box that could cook their food in two minutes without using heat? Would they have been a bit skeptical? Or better yet, what if we took a survey in 1989, and told participants that we had discovered a magic pill that would dramatically increase happiness in marriages? My guess is that people would say "this sounds too good to be true" to all of these ideas, but especially the last one. The point is that sometimes an accidental discovery creates a solution to a problem that we didn't even recognize. In many instances, accidental discoveries are made in one area while trying to solve a problem in a completely unrelated field. This was the case in the discovery of Viagra and was also the case in the discovery of the Sensa Weight-Loss System.

As I mentioned, the biggest objection to dieting is that it causes pain in the form of imposing restrictions and a change of lifestyle habits. The only real pleasure to dieting comes very incrementally during the process after you start to see some results. The pleasure starts to get better with better results but one glaring point remains—the pain is always there. If I was to ask you to design what you felt was the ideal weight loss program, would your answers look something like this?

> "I would be able to enjoy all my favorite foods."
> "I wouldn't have to count calories."
> "I wouldn't have to starve myself."
> "I wouldn't have to eat foods that I don't like."
> "I wouldn't have to take drugs, diuretics or stimulants."
> "The program would be safe."
> "The program would be developed by a doctor."
> "The program would be effective and be backed by clinical testing."
> "The program would be a healthy approach to weight loss."

Congratulations, you have just described the Sensa Weight-Loss Program.

An Accidental, Revolutionary Approach to Weight Loss

What you are about to discover in the chapters ahead is a revolutionary approach to weight loss based on my personal journey as a doctor, eventually arriving at my destination in the field of smell and taste. And just like the accidental discoveries that I mentioned above, you learned that that I also arrived at my destination in the field of smell and taste by accident.

What you are about to experience in this book is your own personal journey—a journey that will bring you to your final destination of a healthier, happier you. You may find that you are like one of the early participants in our clinical study, Marci had already lost and gained more than 600 pounds over a dozen years in diet programs and she was only thirty-two years old. As far as she was concerned, she had wasted years of her life trying to achieve the weight that she would feel happy with. At this point, she was almost 100 pounds overweight and was preparing to make one more attempt to lose those excess pounds and finally be happy. But rather than feeling excited about finally finding a possible new solution to her problem, she became angry and hostile. "So tell me," she said sarcastically, "about all the foods I *can't* have." You will discover how we changed Marci's perception of weight loss forever.

The Program Premises

The Sensa Weight-Loss Program is based on three simple premises:

1. *Feeling Satisfied*—**I truly believe that you will never be successful on any weight loss program unless you enjoy the foods that you eat.** How many times have you said that you are going to begin your diet on Monday and in anticipation of this, you tried to fit in as many of the foods that you love on the weekend. This anticipated deprivation on Monday caused you to overeat and binge Friday, Saturday and Sunday. Sensa allows you to enjoy all of your favorite foods and still lose weight.

2. *Minimal Changes to Your Lifestyle* — Change is one of the most difficult things we experience in life. As humans, we have a built-in, personal comfort zone, and once we deviate from it, we become uneasy and anxious. Our bodies do everything in their power to get back to and maintain that comfort zone. **Anytime a weight-loss program imposes dramatic changes on your lifestyle, it will fail.** Can you identify with any of the following statements in starting a diet program in the past?

"I have to remember to log everything I eat into a journal."
"I have to weigh my portions."
"I have to count calories."
"I have to have grapefruit with every meal."
"I have to, I have to, I have to."

Pretty soon the "have to's" become the "I forgot to's" and eventually turn into "I don't want to's." Sensa works because it is not a diet. Diets restrict and impose a whole host of dramatic changes to your lifestyle. The Sensa Weight-Loss Program introduces a minimal amount of change gradually, thus allowing you to maintain your current lifestyle and still lose weight. The Sensa premise is to be the easiest, simplest way to lose weight.

3. *Safe and Effective* — **Everyone should be concerned about what they put in their bodies. There are numerous weight loss products in the marketplace that have questionable ingredients. In addition to this, before investing in any program, you should research how effective the program has been proven to be.** There are so many programs that claim to

be effective but have no underlying clinical proof. Sensa does not contain any harmful ingredients and has been clinically proven to be effective as determined by a double-blind placebo study conducted by an independent, third-party laboratory.

Program Goals

The overall goal of the Sensa Weight-Loss Program is threefold:

1. To achieve your personal, ideal weight
2. To achieve a healthier lifestyle
3. To provide you with the tools necessary to maintain your ideal weight

The 3 Levels of the Program

In order to achieve this, the program has been designed in three levels. Level 1 is designed as the primary system. Levels 2 and 3 are designed to help you maximize the results and achieve a healthier lifestyle. The three levels are customizable to your individual lifestyle. You decide when to advance to the next level in the program.

Level 1—The Sensa Tastant System

The use of the Sensa Tastant System was created to kick start your weight loss. This system allows you to eat all of your favorite foods, lose weight, and doesn't require any change in your lifestyle. The clinical studies have shown that just the use of these Tastants alone can result in a healthy weight loss of 1 to 2 pounds per week, which is the recommended weight loss pace as specified by many medical organizations. This realistic pace will also result in a more sustainable weight loss.

Level 2—The Sensa Satiety System

The Sensa Satiety System will introduce you to enjoyable foods that will keep you full for a longer period of time. You will learn, for example, that even though a banana and an orange are roughly the same amount of calories, the orange will keep you full longer, and therefore, is a better choice. We have also created a list of Sensa Satiety recipes and a menu plan that will help to increase your level of success on the program.

Level 3—The Sensa Fastercise System

The Sensa Fastercise System is a new approach to exercise. With our busy lifestyles, people find it difficult to carve out time to exercise. This section will introduce you to a gradual program of efficient ways to exercise at home without equipment that will maximize your weight loss and lead you to a healthier lifestyle.

Sensa is designed as a six-month program to achieve the goals mentioned. Whether you decide to perform all the levels of the program at once or gradually introduce them to your lifestyle is up to you. The program was designed to keep change and disruption to your life at a minimum and to be customizable for you individually. I equate it to the nicotine patch program that has been effectively used to help people eliminate the habit of smoking. If you speak to smokers or former smokers, the addiction to smoking is one of the most difficult habits to break. Going "cold turkey" is not necessarily the best answer to breaking the habit because it imposes a sudden, dramatic change to the smoker's life. The nicotine patch program is composed of various levels as well. By using the patch, the smoker is introduced to a gradual reduction in the levels of nicotine that they receive and thus the impact to the smoker's system is minimized over a period of time. Once a minimal level of nicotine has been reached, the next step is to eliminate the habit completely. But just like the Sensa Program, the users decide when to advance to the next level.

The Sensa Weight-Loss Program operates in a very similar fashion. The program introduces you to gradual changes and improvements over time. These changes will eventually become second nature to you. As you work through the program, you will arrive at your final destination of a healthier, happier, thinner you. Not only will you meet your goals, but they will also be easily maintained. My first step in this quest is to provide you with a good understanding of the magnitude of the problem that you are dealing with—the rampant rise of weight gain in this country and throughout the world.

Chapter 2

THE RAMPANT RISE
OF WEIGHT GAIN

It's April 2009, and a young boy named Édgar Enrique Hernández suffered a bout of flu in La Gloria, Mexico, found to be the swine flu, also known as H1N1. Immediately after the outbreak, the Center for Disease Control (CDC) started working with drug companies to get them the materials that they needed to produce a drug to combat the problem.[1] Right after the first report, thousands of miles away in Cairo, Egyptian officials ordered the slaughtering of 300,000 pigs citing that they felt that pigs are the cause of the epidemic. Asian nations activated thermal scanners that were used during the 2003 SARS crisis to check for signs of fever in passengers traveling from North America. In Australia, pilots were not allowed to land unless they reported if there were any passengers with flu-like symptoms aboard. Students at a Chicago school were told not to shake hands with anyone. The European Union's Health Commissioner urged Europeans not to travel to parts of the United States unless it was essential. Pharmacies in Manhattan reported that they couldn't keep paper face masks in stock. At the end of April, a United Airlines Flight with 245 passengers traveling from Munich to Washington, D.C. landed in Boston instead because a passenger had flu symptoms and the airline thought that she required attention.[2] And in New Mexico, which had no reported cases, health officials were so besieged with calls that they had to establish a hot line. Approximately one month after the first reported outbreak, the World Health Organization had confirmed a global tally of 1,490 cases of this "Swine Flu" with 30 deaths, all but one of them in Mexico. The official statement was 30 deaths caused by swine flu.

The Invisible Epidemic

Let's examine another epidemic. Let's first look at the statistics.

- More than 1 billion adults have this disease globally
- More than 31% of U.S. adults have this disease
- Since 1960, this disease has more than doubled among U.S. adults
- More than 17% of U.S. children and adolescents have this disease[3]
- More than 300,000 U.S. adults die from this disease every year[4]

What is this disease? If you guessed obesity, you were correct. We're surrounded by it. We constantly hear it in the news and see it with our own eyes—Americans are larger and heavier than ever before. Obesity is modern society's invisible epidemic and authorities view

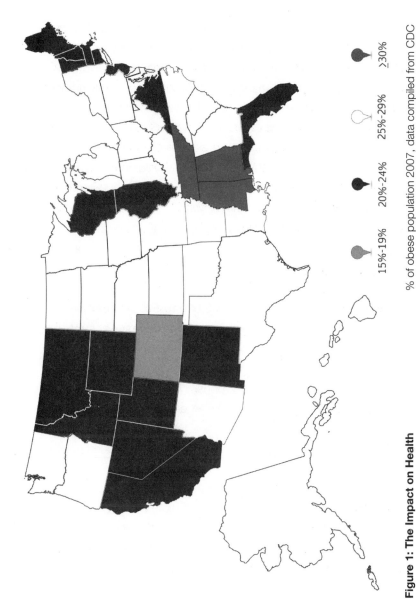

Figure 1: The Impact on Health

15%-19% 20%-24% 25%-29% ≥30%

% of obese population 2007, data compiled from CDC

it as one of the most serious health problems of the 21st century.[5] **According to the World Health Organization, there are over 1 billion adults, about one-sixth of the world's population that are overweight with at least 300 million of them being classified as clinically obese.**[6] This epidemic is not restricted to industrialized societies. The increase in the rate of obesity is growing even faster in developing countries than in the developed world.[7]

More than 60 million adults and 9 million children are classified as obese in the United States. Figure 1 shows the percentage of the population by state in the United States that were classified as obese in 2007. Only one state, Colorado had a prevalence of obesity less than 20%. Thirty states had a prevalence equal to or greater than 25%; three of these states, Alabama, Mississippi and Tennessee, had a prevalence of obesity equal to or greater than 30%.[8]

Every year, anywhere from 300,000 to 500,000 people die in the United States from weight-related illnesses, such as heart attacks, strokes, and cardiovascular or other diseases. In the U.S., obesity is the number two factor as the leading contributor to the cause of death.[9] Clearly, obesity kills.

Children are becoming obese at an earlier age and this trend continues into adulthood. The real problem is that obesity is an evolving disease and the medical effects take time to accumulate. Doctors are seeing Type II diabetes and other weight-related illnesses occurring at a much earlier age.

The difference between the world's reaction to the swine flu epidemic and the epidemic of obesity is interesting to note. At the time of publication, approximately 700 deaths from the H1N1 virus had been reported. The Swine Flu epidemic put people in a panic mode.

Swine flu is a serious epidemic, but to put it into perspective, obesity kills more than 300,000 people annually in this country alone yet it seems that it has taken a back seat position in people's minds. That's why I call it the invisible epidemic.

In relating to the Pleasure/Pain Principle, swine flu causes immediate pain when it is acquired through illness and suffering with absolutely no pleasure attached. The public's reaction was to eliminate the pain or the possibility of pain before it began. The development of an obese condition, on the other hand, has a great amount of pleasure attached to it in the form of satisfying and delicious foods. The pain of obesity, both psychological and physical, takes time to accumulate. It's only at the point when the pain from the disease is greater than the pleasure that comes from eating food that people react and want to make changes in their own lives. Unfortunately, at that point, it is much more difficult to solve the problem.

Furthermore, I don't think that people equate obesity with a disease that has the consequence of death. Thousands of Americans die from this epidemic everyday, but obesity is not classified as a cause-related disease. The coroner will not list "obesity" on the death certificate but rather such things as "cardiac arrest due to coronary artery atherosclerosis." It is very similar to diseases caused by smoking. Although smoking causes death, it is never listed as the cause. Even the warnings on cigarette packs state such things as the following:

"SURGEON GENERAL'S WARNING: Smoking Causes Lung Cancer, Heart Disease, Emphysema, And May Complicate Pregnancy."

Moreover, the cure for swine flu is much more easily attained by developing a flu drug using the strain of flu itself. The disease of obesity is a far more complex one. There has been "no magic pill" developed where after taking it, 50 pounds of overweight fat would immediately be released from the body. There are only a few prescription drugs that have been developed to date and even these have not had much degree of success.

Nothing concerns me more than the statistics mentioned regarding the alarming rate of obesity, not only in this country but around the world. It is a problem that has both physical and psychological consequences, such as social discrimination, low self-esteem and even suicide. The University of Texas has conducted obesity research and in one study found that obese girls are half as likely to attend college as thin girls. The study was composed of 11,000 adolescents and also found that obesity had no impact on college attendance for boys. In addition, obese girls are far more likely to consider suicide and turn to drugs and alcohol than their slimmer counterparts.[10] Clearly, the social implications of self-image for girls are far greater than boys.

To better understand this problem, we can look at the most widely accepted definitions of the terms "overweight" and "obese."

Body Mass Index (BMI)

The Body Mass Index (BMI) is a measurement scale that was actually developed in the 19th century by the Belgian statistician, Adolphe Quetelet. It is a scale that researchers, health professionals and the World Health Organization (WHO) use to estimate the amount of excess weight in the body. The BMI has been used in studies that look for associations between weight and diseases such as diabetes and high blood pressure. As a person's BMI increases above a certain level, so does an individual's risk for developing certain diseases. Not everyone with a high BMI is at risk. Bodybuilders and highly trained athletes are the exception. Although they tend to weigh more, they also have more muscle than fat.

The medical definition of overweight vs. obese depends greatly on the Body Mass Index. BMIs have six categories:

- If your BMI is less than 18.5, it falls within the "underweight" range.
- If your BMI is 18.5 to 24.9, it falls within the "normal" or "healthy" weight range.
- If your BMI is 25 to 29.9, it falls within the "overweight" range.
- If your BMI is 30 or higher, it falls within the "obese" range and is considered Class I obesity.
- If your BMI is 35 to 39.9, it falls within the Class II obesity range.
- If your BMI is 40 or greater, it falls within the Class III obesity range.

How to Calculate BMI

BMI can be calculated easily just using your height and weight. The formula for calculating BMI is as follows:

Weight (in pounds) x 703 ÷ Height (in inches) ÷ Height (in inches) = BMI

For example, let's look at a person who is 5'5" tall (65 inches) and weighs 180 pounds. The formula to calculate BMI would be as follows:

$$180 \times 703 = 126{,}540$$
$$126{,}540 \div 65 = 1946.76$$
$$1946.76 \div 65 = 29.95$$

This person's BMI is 29.95 and this would put them in the "overweight" category. If you don't want to take the time to do the math yourself, you can just go to www.cdc.gov and type in "Adult BMI Calculator" in the site's search field. You will be asked to enter your height and weight. After you have done this, press calculate. Your BMI and the corresponding weight status category will appear.

While the BMI calculator puts the statistics in black and white, let's face it—you probably already know if you're overweight. But it is still a good measurement and goal device to use on your quest to lose weight. You should also take pleasure in seeing yourself lowering your BMI category.

The Roller Coaster

Maybe you woke up one morning, tried to put on your favorite pants and it hit you—"I need to lose weight." Or your twentieth high school reunion is coming up and you want to lose the one-pound-a-year that you've gained since then to get back to your eighteen-year-old waist size. You may have noticed that it's harder to run after your grandchildren since you've put on some weight. You may know that you're 30 pounds overweight and you're embarrassed that every time you lose ten pounds, they seem to come back overnight. Why do you make a conscious decision at certain points in your life to lose weight?

During your weight gain period, the pleasure of eating was far greater than the pain of gaining pounds and being overweight until you reached a determining pain point. This pain point could have taken the form of getting on the scale one day and being overwhelmed by the number you saw, not being able to fit into one of your favorite outfits, or even meeting a friend that you haven't seen for a long time and noticing how much weight he or she has lost. At this point, the pain of that moment was far greater than the pleasure you would receive from eating your favorite foods. This pain caused you to take action to lose weight. And even though the actions that you deemed necessary in the form of pain such as exercise, deprivation and changing your lifestyle were great, the pain of being overweight was greater.

What happens next? You start dieting and you lose a few pounds. You feel better about yourself and you are able to get back into that favorite outfit. Now the pain of being overweight is gone and the pleasure of eating your favorite foods kicks in and you are back to gaining the weight. This roller coaster ride will continue over and over again. But here's the inevitable conclusion. **As you get older, it is more difficult to lose weight because your metabolism slows down.** The roller coaster took the form of gaining and losing weight over the years and it is increasingly more difficult to get back to your "starting" weight. You eventually wake up when you turn 50 and you're 50 pounds overweight. Losing 50 pounds is a lot more difficult than losing 10 pounds. Eventually, at some point, you'll throw up your hands and say, "I give up. I'm never going to diet again." You've gone from being slim to being overweight to being obese, a medical condition with serious and often dire consequences and the clock starts ticking faster toward the medical consequences associated with this devastating disease.

The movie, Wall-E™ depicted the society of the future with people being so obese that they were not able to even walk. They were transported around all day in personal hovercrafts with personal television screens, being served food all day by a robotic population. There was virtually no work for them to do because all the work was conducted by robots. In my opinion, this is not very far from the truth due to the levels of obesity today, the rampant rise of this epidemic as seen over the last 50 years and the fact that this trend will probably continue into the foreseeable future. Couple this with the rise of technological advancements in society today and you have a real Wall-E™ situation. The Director, Andrew Stanton, made a frighteningly accurate prediction of the future and we should view this as a wake-up call for society as a whole.

As you can clearly see, our society is gaining weight at a rapid pace, yet we scrutinize ourselves and others for carrying around the extra pounds. And while we may hold some of the tools to help fight this debilitating disease, you need to understand that your weight gain isn't totally your fault. Changing factors in society and nature have continued to cause the spread of weight gain across the country and the globe.

On your journey to achieve your ideal weight, there is one major enemy to contend with—the natural prevalence in today's society for humans to gain weight. In my work, I see the devastating impact that this enemy has on people. They persecute themselves and blame themselves for being overweight and obese. As you will see in the next chapter, this is as wrong as someone blaming themselves for developing cancer.

Chapter 3

DON'T BLAME YOURSELF FOR BEING OVERWEIGHT

Although weight gain and obesity affect people's physical health, it also affects them psychologically and socially. The devastating effects of depression and social isolation that accompanies obesity aren't as well known. **According to a study led by Sarah M. Markowitz, M.S. (March 2008, Clinical Psychology: Science and Practice), "people who are obese may be more likely to become depressed because they experience themselves as in poor health and are dissatisfied with their appearance."** Generally speaking, our society views overweight people as lazy, stupid, and repugnant while thin people are seen as hard workers, smarter, and more acceptable in every way. Films such as *Norbit* and *Shallow Hal* may have overweight people as their main characters (or thin people disguised as overweight people), but we are meant to laugh at them and their size. There was even a recent study conducted that blames "fat" people for global warming.[11]

Even medical professionals treat their overweight patients with less respect than their average-sized patients. Studies show that doctors spend more time with thin patients than those who are overweight and are likely to respond to thin people in a more positive way. If a thin person and an overweight individual are interviewed for the same position, the thin person is more likely to get the job.

What is harder to quantify is the extent to which being overweight impacts social interaction. Overweight people can be reluctant to leave the house and often avoid social events. Internalizing society's view of obesity, overweight people think of themselves as inferior to people of average weight. They are less assertive in social situations, on the job, or in academic arenas. Their negative feelings reflect on their interactions with their spouses and other family members, which in turn, affect the behavior of everyone around them.

A disturbing dichotomy exists between the medical model of obesity—a disease—and the social model of obesity as a weak character trait indicative of laziness. In our politically correct environment, people wouldn't dream of ostracizing someone with diabetes or cancer, yet somehow it's okay to do so to a larger person. Society assumes that obese people are incompetent, lazy, and self-indulgent. Its anger towards them exceeds any rational approach. Rather than being empathetic, people are annoyed with larger people. Why? They fear that if they were to lose control of their will power, they too could end up overweight.

Our attitude is not based on the desire to see health in our fellow humans, but instead is emotionally driven. It's a result of internal ambivalence regarding our own self-control. The obese person is a physical representation of the lack of control lurking within our-selves, and therefore, we assign a negative connotation to them. We fear them and tease them in an attempt to marginalize them so they are no longer in our consciousness. And at the same time we try to make ourselves seem superior. Regardless of whether obesity is of a genetic origin, situational, or disease-related, our response to the obese is prejudice.

Three-quarters of all girls and half of all boys in college say they have been on a diet or managed their food intake for the purpose of losing weight. Everywhere you look, there are weight-loss books and websites, ads for by-pass surgery, and costly diet programs that promise to tame the obesity monster.

The obesity epidemic is spreading throughout the world as other cultures and countries adopt Western food patterns of eating fast food, drinking sugary beverages, and snacking between meals.

Why Do We Eat So Much?

The amount of food we consume has grown at a frightening level, along with our waistlines and risk for serious disease. **The per capita, daily calorie consumption (PCDCC) in the United States increased from 2234 in 1970 to 2757 in 2003, an increase of 23.4%.**[12] In order to put this in perspective, we need to take a look at a measurement known as the basal metabolic rate. This rate measures the calorie consumption of our bodies in a fully rested position on a daily basis. A "calorie" is a measurement of energy for our bodies just as a "watt" is a measure of energy for electricity.

It is a generally known fact that if we consume more calories in the form of food than calories that we expend on a daily basis through activities, we will gain weight over time since our bodies store this excess energy in the form of fat. If we expend more energy than we ingest, then over time we will lose weight. But how do we determine this? How do we know how much energy our own bodies need to expend on a daily basis to determine this? As a starting point, we need to understand that our bodies need a certain amount of calorie consumption just to remain sedentary each day, which is equivalent to lying in bed and not moving for an entire 24 hour period. The reason for this is that our various organs and bodily functions such as breathing require energy. The amount of energy needed for this is called our Basal Metabolic Rate and is different for every person. The rate is based on gender, height, weight, and age. You can search online for "basal metabolic rate" and numerous sites will come up where you can enter your own data to calculate your own personal BMR. Let's look at an example.

A male who is 40 years old, 5'9" tall, and who weighs 180 pounds has a BMR of 1792 which means that his body will burn 1792 calories just by lying in bed for 24 hours or remaining sedentary. If you deduct the above BMR from the U.S. per capita daily consumption of calories (PCDCC) shown above, you get the following equation:

2757 (PCDCC) — 1792 (BMR of 40 year old above) =
965 excess calories

One pound of weight gain or loss is equivalent to 3500 calories.[13] So, we would have to ingest or expend 3500 excess calories above our daily caloric needs in order to gain or lose 1 pound on the scale. In the current example, if this person lies in bed all day, every day, and someone just fed him the per capita American daily consumption of calories (2757), he would take in roughly 6755 more calories per week than he needs as shown in the following calculation:

965 (daily excess calories) x 7 (days per week) = 6755 (excess calories)

If he did nothing but lay in bed for an entire year, then he would gain an average of 1.93 pounds per week (6755 divided by 3500), or more than 100 pounds during the year. Although this may sound like a ridiculous example, I have seen many examples of people in the news who weigh 500, 600, and even 800 pounds who have to lie in bed all day because they can't get up and move. In some cases, the use of a crane has had to be used to remove them from the house in order to treat a medical condition in a hospital. Obviously, the above calculation is an extreme example since most people expend additional energy (calories) in various activities during the day. As a whole, our society today is ingesting more calories in food than we are expending in energy and that is the basic reason for the dramatic rise in the number of overweight and obese people.

But as you will see, our society has changed and there are a number of new factors that have arisen that have negatively affected our ability to maintain a healthy weight. You need to understand them in order to come to the realization that there are many forces operating against you. In some cases, you have the ability to overcome them. The trends that you will see are due to changes that have impacted society over the last ten, twenty, fifty and one hundred years. Newton observed that every action has an equal and opposite reaction. The actions that have taken place during this period have dramatically impaired our ability to control our weight.

Sedentary Lifestyle

As a society over the last decade, we have become more sedentary in our daily lifestyles. I believe that this is largely due to both our changing work environments and the amount of non-physical, technological entertainment at our disposal today. It's been found that 40% of adults in the United States do not participate in any form of leisure time physical activity.[14] With all of the increased non-physical, indoor entertainment options being developed today, it should be no surprise that we are spending less and less time enjoying outdoor physical activities. These options have even impaired the outdoor physical activities of our children and adolescents. In a recent study, researchers found that 89% of so-called physical activities by three- to five-year-olds were found to be sedentary at community-based preschool programs, as were more than half of their outdoor activities.[15] It's been determined that 43% of adolescents watch more than 2 hours of television per day.[16] With the advent of computers and video games, children and adolescents spend more and more time in front of entertainment screens without physical activities Even in adults, the computer and television has taken over a great deal of our lives. A recent trend shows that the internet is infringing on television usage, but the aspect of sitting idly in front of any screen for hours at a time both at work and at home connotes an expenditure of less caloric activity in our daily life.

More and more people live in suburbs and other communities where they have to drive everywhere. Unlike urban living, where you can walk a block or two to get a quart of milk or a bit further to go to the gym, those who live in suburban communities use their cars to travel everywhere—often just a few blocks—so they are walking far less than city dwellers. Television, video games, and other solitary endeavors keep us in the house and on the couch. And what comes with this sedentary activity? Eating more food. Today, food and television go hand-in-hand. One of the biggest national American parties is centered on watching the Super Bowl and consuming large amounts of food and alcohol. Grocery stores actively promote this event and increase their inventory levels to meet the needs for that celebrated Sunday.

Higher Caloric Values in Food

With the advent of the trends of two income households, people marrying at a later age and more single households, Americans are preparing less and less meals from scratch and relying more and more on fast and processed foods. These foods traditionally have higher caloric value, ounce vs. ounce, than unprocessed foods such as fruits and vegetables. In addition, according to Dr. Richard Wrangham, an anthropologist from Harvard University, a much higher percentage of softer, processed foods get absorbed into our system than harder unprocessed foods. This increases the percentage of calories that enter our systems dramatically.[17] In fact, Dr. Wrangham believes that the rise of processed foods is the number one cause of the modern epidemic of obesity. Our reliance on these foods has caused us to ingest a much higher degree of calories than our bodies need on a daily basis. In addition, there is one food ingredient that could be playing a major role in the obesity epidemic not only in America but around the world.

High Fructose Corn Syrup (HFCS)

The consumption of high fructose corn syrup has skyrocketed in this country, increasing 1000% between 1970 and 1990.[18] Due to cost factors, company after company has replaced traditional sweetening ingredients with HFCS, which now represents more than 40% of caloric sweeteners added to foods. It is also the sole ingredient used as a sweetening agent in non-diet soft drinks in the United States.[19] The problem with this is that the body processes HFCS in a different manner than traditional sweetening agents. The digestion, absorption, and metabolism of HFCS are different than traditional glucose. HFCS is not very effective in stimulating insulin secretion or enhancing leptin production which act as key afferent signals in the regulation of food intake and body weight.[20] The continued increase of consumption of soft drinks could play a major role in inducing increased consumption of calories from other foods as well.

Larger Food Portion Sizes

There are many reasons why we're eating more food and packing on the pounds. Portion sizes in restaurants and at home have become enormous. They are 3 times larger today than they were 25 years ago. Ask any restaurateur and he'll tell you that if he cuts the amount of food that he serves, his patrons will complain that they're not getting their money's worth. As children, we have been told to eat everything on our plates, and with the advent of these larger portion sizes, we tend to consume more food and more calories.

When it comes right down to it, the bottom line is that we're making poor choices and we're never satisfied. How is that possible? We're never satisfied because the food we eat has little real flavor or taste. The worst part is that the increase in calorie consumption is accompanied by an increase in the amount of sedentary lifestyles, mentioned before, so there's no additional expenditure of energy to work off those additional calories.

Climate Controlled Environments

Today, we live in a society where our everyday existence is housed in air conditioned and heated surroundings. Our ancestors were used to either shivering or sweating in their daily lives before the advent of climate regulating machines. As you probably realize, shivering and sweating actually use up body energy and thus expend calories. Not only this, but in society today, our bodies go from one mini-climate-controlled environment to the next. We live in our climate-controlled homes, get into our climate-controlled cars, work in our climate-controlled offices, and shop in our climate-controlled stores. Even many factory environments today are climate-controlled. As a society, we have come to expect perfect, personal, climatic conditions. People even complain today if the temperature of the room that they are in is a few degrees warmer or colder than they would like.

Higher Levels of Pollution

Believe it or not, the rising levels of pollution in our society may increase body weight and lead to obesity. **A groundbreaking study from Spain conducted in 2008 suggests that pollution exposure for mothers may increase their baby's propensity for obesity as they get older.**[21] Although the study measured the effects of just one pollutant, a pesticide, the study shows that exposure to the hundreds of pollutants we encounter on a daily basis may contribute to obesity in both children and in adults.

Prescription Drugs

Today, as a society, we have become very dependent on prescription drugs. The retail sales of these products in the United States hit over $286 billion in 2007.[22] The drug companies have even taken to the television airwaves to promote their individual drugs to solve all of your problems. As we all know, drugs can have many side effects and certain drugs such as contraceptives, steroid hormones, some antidepressants, and blood pressure drugs can cause weight gain.[23]

Lack of Sleep

"America is becoming a sleep deprived nation" according to researcher, Denise Amschler. With our busier schedules, more and more people are suffering from lack of sleep. **In research conducted by U.S. scientists in conjunction with researchers at the University of Bristol, lack of sleep could lead to hormonal changes that increase appetite.**[24] The study found that less sleep produces more of the hormone, grehlin, which increases appetite, and less of the hormone, leptin which suppresses appetite.

As you have read, our society has dramatically changed. Due to numerous factors, our lifestyles have been forever altered and the consequences have been devastating to our health. The point is, don't persecute yourself for your weight gain. There are more variables against you today than you may have imagined.

Chapter 4

WHY DIETING DOESN'T WORK

Gretchen is 50 years old. She has tried virtually every diet program on the market. Although she has not kept track of how much weight she has lost during her 50 years, she guesses it's in the hundreds of pounds. "I probably could have created two to three new people from the weight that I have lost." Unfortunately, she has gained all the weight back and has experienced a net increase of 50 pounds on her 5'6" frame since she began her first diet when she was 25 and weighed 125. That's a two-pound-a-year increase, about double the national average for weight gain over the years as you age. "No matter what I try, I can't keep the weight off. It comes off for a while but then I just seem to gain it back."

Why do we struggle so much with weight loss? Why is it so difficult to permanently lose weight? Why can't we just maintain the weight we had as a teenager? Millions of people that fail on diets ask themselves these questions every day. Without question, we can say that over the long term, diets almost never work, but the fault may not lie with the dieter. That, it appears, is something that most overweight people don't know. For a partial reason for this, we can look to our evolution.

Million of Years of Evolution

While I don't expect an overweight person to be happy about being a victim of evolution, being afflicted with a problem also means being a survivor in a long evolutionary struggle. I'm talking about millions of years of the human struggle to survive. For much of our history, the quest for survival was a daily concern. Think about it for a minute. When you studied history, did you ever read about a society with not only an abundance of food, but vast stores of *excess* food? You didn't read about such a society because it has never existed before. We are at a unique point in history, and from what we know about human development, this excess of food is actually an unnatural condition.

Most of our ancestors had to accumulate fat in the food growing season in order to survive cold winters, during which they consumed whatever stored food was available, and when they ran out they foraged for more. These were the only available options. Until very recently, it was common for food supplies to dwindle during the cold, winter months, particularly in the Northern Hemisphere. Many people became hungry before winter's end, and spring was greeted with great rejoicing, not just because it was warm and pleasant, but because food supplies could be renewed. It's likely that the spring rituals and festivals originated precisely because new plant and animal life appeared just in time to ensure survival for one more year.

We know it's easier to lose weight in the summer when fat is, in a biological sense, not as necessary because food is available. In the Northern Hemisphere, we developed in a way similar to the black bear; we accumulate fat in the winter as a supplementary source of calories for use when food is scarce.

In the past, periodic famine was not just an occasional threat; it was a regular reality throughout the world. And, during those miserable periods, only those that stored body fat survived. In fact, those, whose bodies could efficiently accumulate fat, were strong enough to flourish to reproduce. This is one of the best examples we can look to that demonstrate the "survival of the fittest." Perhaps when we hear people admire a plump baby, we are also hearing an attitude that has carried over from our evolutionary past. Imagine how relieved new parents were when a baby was born with what at one time was viewed as a positive feature—fat, plenty of fat. Throughout Western literature, we can read descriptions of fat babies and the way this was viewed as a sign of good health and a strong constitution. To be sure, in many places in the world, famine is still a reality that threatens to become even more severe. (Unfortunately, hunger and lack of adequate nutrition is not completely unknown in our own wealthy country either.)

In other countries, food scarcity is more than the distant memory it is to most of us born and raised in this country. Indeed, food is still so scarce in some places that the main occupation of men and women is securing enough of it to stay alive. Edward, one of our study participants, who has struggled with his weight problem for fifty years, described this paradoxical situation well. "When I lived and worked in a number of Asian countries," he said, "older women in the villages admired my big waistline. They thought that I must be prosperous to be so fat. They found Americans fascinating in part because we have those excess pounds. To these women, who had been poor most of their lives, my fat was a sign of good fortune. I was blessed with more than enough food."

While a scant food supply is no longer as pressing an issue in most of the countries Edward worked in, the older people remember the days when famine constantly threatened them. As we've seen in many countries, food shortages always threaten. It goes without saying that people in many other cultures consider our society's obsession with weight as rather odd and even self-indulgent. While it may be small comfort if you live in the image-conscious United States, being very thin is not admired in much of the rest of the world.

Ironically, as soon as Edward moved back to the United States, he embarked on numerous diets and even fasting programs in order to lose his excess pounds. Much of the time, he did lose weight, but within a few months he gained the unwanted pounds back, and more. When he first began his quest to lose weight and tried many diets, he had 45 pounds to lose; when I saw him, that number had grown to more than 100. Predictably, he was unhappy and frustrated.

One African-American woman questioned the premise about fat accumulation in the Northern Hemisphere. After all, she said, her ancestors were not from Europe. Why was she fat? I could tell her only that the distribution of obesity throughout our population suggests that when food becomes plentiful, the evolutionary mandates for survival can lead to excess fat accumulation in all racial groups. This, combined with our society's emphasis on food, sets up a situation in which large numbers of people from all racial and ethnic backgrounds become vulnerable to weight gain. We have seen it takes only a generation or two for weight to become a problem among our immigrant populations.

Fighting Evolution

It's a paradox, but now that the strongest have survived because their ancestors stored fat so efficiently, the problems that new generations face have changed. Many people have bodies that are too efficient, and they have a difficult time adapting to our unique conditions, specifically, abundant food all year round. In other words, for many people, the struggle to survive has been won, and now the struggle to maintain health is in conflict with our innate biological programming. The body simply doesn't know what is going on here. It's as if it's saying, "Wait a minute here. I'm supposed to be storing fat so that you can get through lean periods. But you're eating so much all year round, and I don't know how to turn this storage system off. What do you want from me? My main job is to make sure you survive, but you're confusing me."

Our bodies are incredible machines and are beautifully programmed to maintain homeostasis, that is, to stay the same, to maintain. Again, this is an important evolutionary strength. When food is scarce, the body will slow the metabolic rate in order to "hoard" its available fuel. The brain gets used to, or set at, a certain weight; it struggles to keep the body stabilized at that rate, usually referred to as the "set point."

The "roller coaster" syndrome is the result of the body's fight to maintain homeostasis. If diets worked, then each

41

overweight person would go on one diet in a lifetime and never need to worry about the scale traveling up and down— again and again. But, we're in a situation in which it appears that homeostasis, the evolutionary friend, has now become the dieter's enemy.

It's no wonder that the majority of people in our studies had not only been on numerous self-directed diets, but had also participated in many commercial or employer-sponsored weight loss programs. Astounding as it seems, our participants listed close to one hundred different programs. Every person has been on at least six or seven diets before entering our weight loss program. In almost every case, the weight returned in a relatively short period of time, sometimes within a few months.

The "roller coaster" syndrome is most dramatic among people who fast or who are on very low calorie diets. Some people cut their calorie intake even more during a plateau, which leads to lack of energy and increased hunger. Eventually, most people stop the diet, usually believing that they have failed again. It's difficult enough to lose weight when you feel good, but when you feel physically and emotionally defeated, it is almost impossible.

Women and the Evolutionary Trail

You've no doubt heard women say, "It's so infuriating. He eats one piece of toast instead of two, switches to light beer, cuts his snacks in half, and he loses weight. I practically starve myself to get rid of one lousy pound, and he's boasting about the five pounds he's dropped this week. I can't stand it."

In the interest of the survival of our species, women are clearly important. Much as we men may dislike this, it's a fact that in the natural scheme of things, nature can afford to lose more men than women. Thus, the women who store enough fat to both survive and reproduce are the heartiest among us.

Unfortunately, this biological imperative also makes it difficult for women to lose weight, particularly pre-menopausal women whose fertility must, in the evolutionary sense, be protected. A husband can brag about his weight loss, but in our abundant society, he now has a distinct advantage. The fact that he's more biologically dispensable makes it easier for him to fight evolution. This is one reason that more women are overweight than men.

Estrogen, one of the female hormones responsible for ovulation, also appears to play a part in maintaining weight. Where once this was a blessing, it is now a curse of sorts. Back when food supplies were seasonal and generally scarce, a woman who efficiently maintained body fat could ovulate and carry a fetus to term. Hence, new generations could continue because of women's ability to store fat and because of the body's struggle to maintain homeostasis.

Frankly, our bodies haven't changed much in response to excess food supplies. In our weight loss study, we noted that pre-menopausal women and those on estrogen replacement therapy (ERT), lost weight at a slower rate than men and post-menopausal women who were not taking estrogen. (This difference should not discourage women from attempting to lose weight with the Sensa Program, nor should it prompt them to stop taking estrogen. Many women benefit from ERT in that it may help prevent osteoporosis and symptoms associated with menopause. The relative benefits and risks of ERT should be discussed with your gynecologist.)

The biological situation which works against women, combined with our society's emphasis on being thin, contribute to the continuation of the "roller coaster syndrome"—more diets, more self-help programs, more weight loss centers. And for many people, especially women, this atmosphere finally results in the depressing conclusion that one more diet isn't the answer. And they're right. The answer is the same for men. **Diets simply don't work.**

Life often feels unfair, but nowhere is this more true than in the struggle of weight loss. If you get the feeling that you've been set up to struggle with weight, and that it just doesn't seem fair, you're entirely correct. You may be like some of the more than three thousand people in our weight loss study: you've gained and lost hundreds of pounds in your lifetime; you've suffered the emotional roller coaster that goes along with roller coaster dieting; you've suffered serious consequences, both physical and emotional, from being overweight.

Food Fight

In addition to fighting evolution, you are also up against society's emphasis on food which—co-exists with worshipping thinness, a trend that is especially popular right now. Just think about the food messages that bombard you on a daily basis. There are people who can't stand to watch a pizza television commercial without ordering one; it's as if the smell of the pizza comes right through the screen. Both the sight and smell of food are before us constantly, ever enticing us to eat. "All you can eat" is a watchword of some restaurants and even in some of our homes. We are programmed to think that there is never enough, and more is better. (Of course, this "more is better" mentality affects practically everything from food to the amount of money we make to the size of our homes. It can be a discouraging mind-set; it may feed our competitive drive, but is ultimately demoralizing for many people.)

Food as Comfort

In addition to the temptations that surround us, most overweight people acknowledge that they also use food for comfort. The mere act of eating can relieve stress and inner turmoil. Yet, many of those who are not overweight eat for the same reasons. People in our society joke about eating ice cream when they don't have a date on Saturday night. Or people freely talk about overeating at dinner on the day the big business deal fell through. But, it's usually thin people who discuss this openly. The overweight person often is silent or will attempt to deny that he or she uses food to combat emotional difficulty. They sometimes think of this as a secret shame and only in support groups will they "confess" to overeating and—even binging when they feel sad or hopeless. This emotional connection is one of the major reasons why diets can't work. In today's world, we are subject to many emotional stresses that drive us to seek comfort in food, especially in the ones that we truly enjoy. While eating for emotional reasons has often been viewed as a problem or an emotional disorder, it is nearly a universal phenomenon. Overweight people aren't really that different from their slimmer sisters and brothers.

The vast majority of people have used food for purposes other than to meet nutritional needs. When we were babies, we cried and were offered food for comfort. In some cases we were hungry and in others we weren't. Either way, we associated this offer of food with love and being taken care of. As children, we may have been rewarded with food when we received good grades or for any other number of reasons. Sybil, a participant in our study, told us that her family had an elaborate dinner in an expensive restaurant every time her mother sold one of her paintings. Clearly, food was associated with success. Is it any wonder that now, when Sybil makes important sales for her company, her first impulse is to eat? When she loses a sale, her urge to eat is just as strong. Her emotional response is learned.

Social Pressures to Eat

Martin found that when he was following one of his strict diets, it was difficult to have a social life. Women he dated didn't understand that he wanted to skip dinner and head straight to the movie theater. His dates didn't particularly like it when he didn't want to share a bucket of buttered popcorn, and he preferred not to be tempted at a café where good smelling pastries called out to him from display cases. So ingrained is our association of food with social activity that Martin wound up isolated when he found it too difficult to handle constant temptation. Because diets don't work, Martin went through periods of having a social life, with all the associated meals and treats, and periods of being alone, combined with attempts to lose weight. Believe me; his roller coaster story is not unique.

I've heard people say that they were urged not to begin a diet until after the holidays. After all, how could they enjoy the season between late November and January unless they could eat all of their favorite foods? Others have said that they are afraid of hurting someone's feelings by not taking second helpings.

So, if you are overweight and sense that the cards have been stacked against you, you are right. And as you can see, in addition to having evolutionary factors working to contend with, you also have against you the very society that urges you to eat.

Food Restrictions

Losing weight is a very simple equation. Take in fewer calories than you expend in energy and you will lose weight. Consume more calories than you burn and you will gain weight. If you look at many of the popular diet plans in the marketplace, they mask this equation by imposing unreasonable food restrictions. One plan restricts carbohydrates; another one restricts fats; another restricts proteins. Any one of these diets imposes a dramatic, immediate change in eating habits that is rarely sustainable. At the beginning of the plan, people are motivated due to the pain of weight gain. They start the plan and start to see results. Eventually, the pain of not being able to eat many of their favorite foods is greater than the pleasure of the weight loss that they are experiencing. That is one of the main reasons that people cannot stay on these restrictive plans.

Unrealistic, Unsustainable Weight-Loss Amounts

You've finished the holidays, gained a few pounds and the new year is upon you. It's the perfect time to make a new start in life. That's why everybody loves the start of the new year. It's as if we are all just born again. It's the perfect time for a do-over. We can forget everything bad that has happened this past year, including gaining those unsightly pounds.

It should be no surprise that January is the prime selling season for weight-loss products. Watch any television program in January and you will see promises of fast weight loss in a multitude of advertisements. "Lose 10 pounds in 10 days!" "Frank lost 10 pounds the first week." Are these true? Perhaps. The actual amount of fat lost in this short period of time is probably very little. And these best case scenario examples are often not sustainable due to homeostasis which I discussed earlier. If the body starts to see a dramatic loss in weight in a short period of time, it will react and try to counteract the effect in order to survive. This is why most medical practitioners recommend gradual weight loss of 1–2 pounds per week. Unfortunately, we all want fast results, but just because something is quick does not mean it is long-term.

Over the last few chapters, I hoped that I've shown you how widespread the problem of weight gain has become in society, the consequences of the epidemic and why you should not necessarily blame yourself for your problem. In this chapter, I've shown you the factors against you, including your own body, in trying to lose weight using traditional "dieting" methods. In the next chapters, you will see how you can approach weight loss using a completely new method—how you can use the same body that has been working against you to your benefit in achieving your weight-loss goals.

Chapter 5

THE IMPACT OF
SMELL AND TASTE
ON OUR LIVES

All of our senses are designed to help us survive. We hear sounds that alert us to danger and inform us about situations to help us cope with the world around us. We see things that threaten us and this same sense of sight directs us to a safe place. Our sense of touch alerts us to bodily injury in the form of pain and tells us to either quickly move to avoid further pain or to seek treatment for it. If we didn't have these senses, we would probably have died in infancy. Can you remember the first time that you felt the sensation of fire? These same three senses—sight, touch, and hearing—can also give us great pleasure in the form of listening to great music, viewing a beautiful sunset and enjoying a wonderful massage.

Our other two senses—smell and taste, also act as a survival mechanism and provide us with great pleasure as well. The smell and taste of spoiled food can keep us from poisoning ourselves as well as allow us to enjoy the aroma and flavor of a gourmet meal.

Of the five senses, our sense of smell is probably the most under-rated sense that we use. In fact, we are probably not even aware of how much we use it. It can affect our moods. The smells in a doctor's office can make us anxious. The smells in a coffee shop can wake us up and get us energized to take on the day. It can affect our emotions as when we smell the scent of freshly baked chocolate chip cookies, taking us back to our childhood with mom in the kitchen. The scent of freshly cut evergreens can evoke memories of the holidays. Smell can protect us as when the scent of smoke puts us on alert, or when the scent of burning food makes us run to the kitchen to turn down the burner to avoid a fire. In fact, research today is showing that we are just hitting the tip of the iceberg in the different ways that the sense of smell impacts our lives. It continues to have many more implications than we can imagine.

As the Neurological Director of the Smell & Taste Treatment and Research Foundation in Chicago, I began uncovering important clues into the underlying mechanisms of hunger and appetite. Over the course of twenty-five years, I have conducted ongoing studies on the effects of smell and taste on eating habits, as well as how smells effect perception of age and weight, the size of a room, and even anxiety or peacefulness. My decades of research have shown that the sense of smell is an important influence on human behavior, emotions, and perception. What follows in this chapter are some real life examples of the effect of smell on everyday life, and how these many implications started to form the key in my mind to unlock the power of how your nose can help you lose weight without dieting.

"Only the Nose Knows"

Have you ever been around a smell that really bothered you? About ten years ago, I received a call from a thirty-year-old Miami woman who could barely tolerate being in the presence of any aroma. The proximity of the aroma to her location made very little difference. All smells were too much for her to handle without becoming sick. She suffered from an extremely oversensitive sense of smell. Throughout my work I have seen such hypersensitivity in many patients. In our field we call this Multiple Chemical Sensitivity, or MCS. MCS is diagnosed when a patient is anxious and uncomfortable due to smell. There's also an increase in sweating and heart rate, and the condition is often associated with dizziness, confusion, and feeling ill. In the past, when my colleagues and I have studied patients who have been diagnosed with MCS, we have found that while odors may cause the problem, it requires a conscious recognition of those odors for the problem to occur. For example, we took patients who had been diagnosed with MCS and placed them in a booth in our laboratory. In our first test we infused the booth with a peppermint aroma—a smell that we already knew had no effect on the patients. In our second test, we replaced the smell of peppermint with the scent of a petroleum substance which we knew had a negative effect on the patients in the past. The petroleum smell caused an increase in heart rate for the patients, as well as dizziness and discomfort. To further our test, we took the same patients and placed them back into the booth. This time we included both the petroleum substance and peppermint, but we made certain the peppermint aroma was more noticeable so that the patient was not conscious of the petroleum smell. All of the patients, mostly women, had no reaction. The result suggested they had to consciously recognize the smell of the petroleum for it to have an effect. The results of the study provided me with two successful treatment options for my patient from Miami. I could either treat her by masking odors to reduce her symptoms or alternatively, recommend the use of medications to affect her sense of smell.

Have you ever been in a situation where you could smell something that a friend couldn't? In another case, my colleagues and I had the opportunity to study a woman from Florida who contacted us about the problems she was experiencing due to her hypersensitivity to aromas. My initial reaction was that she probably had MCS as well. But, when we tested her, what we found was startling. During our first phone conversation, the young woman claimed to have a better-than-normal sense of smell. To give you a better idea of what she experienced, it was as if she could see in color and the rest of the human population could see in just black and white. Our tests showed that she actually did have a better-than-normal sense of smell. In fact, we concluded that her sense of smell was about 100,000 times better than the average person. While you may think her problem doesn't sound like a problem at all, what it really meant was that her hypersensitivity to smells, aromas, and odors caused her to become agoraphobic. I am sure you have heard on television or have read in a magazine about people who have a fear of going outside or being in any open space. That is medically known as agoraphobia. The young lady's overwhelming sense of smell kept her from living a normal life because she had such a fear of leaving her home. In fact, my colleagues and I spent an enormous amount of time trying to convince her to fly to the clinic in Chicago so that we could study her. She was finally able to fly with the use of a face mask.

After a series of additional tests, we found that she had adrenal cortical deficiency, or Addison's disease, the same illness from which President Kennedy suffered. My medical colleagues at the Mayo Clinic, which is known for its practice dedicated to the diagnosis and treatment of just about every kind of complex illness, describes Addison's disease as a disorder that is the result of insufficient production of certain hormones from your adrenal glands. Addison's disease can occur at any age, but is most common in people ages thirty to fifty. Knowing that Addison's disease can be life-threatening, we treated her with adrenal cortical steroids and her sense of smell returned to normal.

While the above examples may seem very atypical and clinical, I hope that you are able to get a clear idea of how important the sense of smell is to human behavior and how we, at our foundation, use over-sensitivity to smells or the loss of smell to help patients with an array of medical conditions. These treatments give us tremendous insight into both the problems and the possibilities that the senses of smell and taste provide.

Now that we have discussed smell-related issues, let's explore some interesting ways in which you can take advantage of your sense of smell.

"Honey, Do These Jeans Make Me Look Fat?"

How many times have you heard or spoken this phrase? You may want to spray a fragrance in the room before you ask your "honey" that particular question. It's true! **Certain aromas can change the perception of a person's weight, and even a person's age.**

In 2007, my colleagues and I studied the effects of odorants on men's perception of a woman's weight. We asked a 245–pound female model to wear a floral-spice fragrance and tested the response of 199 males. We compared this test group to a control group where the model was not wearing any fragrance. The results showed that compared to the non-odorant control group, the floral-spice fragrance reduced the men's perception of the woman's weight by 4.1 pounds. In the males who actually found the floral smell pleasing to their nose, the reduction in weight was 12 pounds. The conclusion was that wearing a floral-spice fragrance can reduce a woman's perceived weight by as much as 5%.

The following year our research uncovered a fact that a certain scent had a rejuvenating affect on the perception of age. The models in the study, when viewed by men and women with that scent present, were estimated to be as much as three years younger when compared to the estimation without the smell present.

If you believe the above studies have very little to no affect on your everyday life, think about the multi-billion dollar business of perfumes and colognes that are sold at some of your favorite department stores, and the aromatherapy and anti-aging products that you can find at every bath and body store. The average person buys these items to feel and look his or her best. For every individual, "looking his or her best" may mean something different. For some people a new perfume or cologne may help them feel prettier, younger, or happier. My point here is that, once again, your nose and your sense of smell play a powerful role in your daily life.

Follow Your Nose

In one of our more recent studies, we found that when people exercise in the presence of buttered popcorn or strawberries, they actually burn more calories in the same time period than if no popcorn or strawberries were present. You'll find that you can burn almost 20 percent more calories. Why? Our studies have shown that the scents of buttered popcorn and strawberry aid in keeping your mind off of the actual act of exercising while keeping you more awake and alert. An increase in alertness while doing physical activities can give you added energy and increase momentum. The more energy you have, the less fatigued you feel while exercising. So if you are in the gym and want to burn more calories, put some buttered popcorn or strawberries nearby (if allowed) to see if it helps your focus—just try not to eat them!

Smell vs. Taste

Food . . . the sight of it, the smell of it and the taste of it can give you a real sense of joy. **Did you know that approximately 90% of what you may refer to as taste is really smell?** Have you ever noticed that when you have come down with a terrible cold and you can't smell anything that you can't taste anything either? But, the minute you can smell that chicken soup, you can also taste it.

I want you to conduct an experiment. Have someone cut up an onion and an apple into similar size pieces. Now, close your eyes and hold your nose tightly so that you can't smell and have him/her feed you each item without telling you which one is which. Can you distinguish which one was the apple and which one was the onion?

They may seem indistinguishable. Without your sense of smell, it is nearly impossible to taste the difference. This is a form of synesthesia, a misperception of one sense for another. Commonly, when you refer to taste, it is really smell.

Odorants and aromas that come from outside the nose, into the nose to the top of the nose are called smells. On the other hand, odorants and aromas from food that come from the mouth and travel up the back of the throat through the top of the nose are called taste.

If this is true, then can the craving for a food be satisfied just by smelling it rather than eating it? If you were to place the smell of chocolate in a bottle to carry around all day and sniff at your leisure, would you still need to eat that chocolate to feel satisfied? If the craving could be eliminated just by smelling the scent of a food, then could this action help us to control appetite and thus help you consume fewer calories? The answer to this question along with something called Sensory Specific Satiety, was paramount in unlocking the door to a completely new way of approaching weight control.

Chapter 6

SENSORY SPECIFIC SATIETY

It's a Friday night and you are sitting around with friends and family for an enjoyable night in. Everyone is hungry and pepperoni pizza sounds perfect. As the delivery boy shows up, the smell of the pizza wafts through the room and the hunger intensifies. Everyone eats their first slice...second slice...maybe even a third. Soon the aroma of the pepperoni pizza that caused your mouths to drool twenty minutes ago doesn't smell as appealing anymore. You remove the pizza box from the room because just the smell is enough to make your feelings of fullness intensify. Someone comes in the room and asks, "Who wants some chocolate chip ice cream?" Everyone raises a hand. Yet, even after everyone has had his or her fill of pizza, there is still room for a serving of ice cream. What's the reason for this?

It's called **Sensory Specific Satiety—the feeling of fullness or satiety that we experience for each specific food as we eat it.** Barbara Rolls from Johns Hopkins University School of Medicine pioneered the concept of Sensory Specific Satiety by testing subjects who initially tasted and rated their enjoyment of eight different foods. After the rating, they ate as much as they wanted of *one* of the foods and then rated the same eight foods again. The pleasantness rating of the one food that was eaten decreased more substantially than the pleasantness rating of the foods that were not eaten. Sensory Specific Satiety is somewhat complex and is influenced by a number of different factors of food—taste, aroma, shape, texture and other sensory properties. This state involves three specific senses—sight (shape), taste (flavor, texture), and smell (aroma).

Evolutionary Reasons for Sensory-Specific Satiety

In theory, Sensory Specific Satiety may have substantial survival value. By eating many different foods with different nutritional components and by varying your diet, you would get all the nutrition you need. So, instead of eating all of the same foods over and over again, primitive man would be driven to eat many different types of food, thereby expanding nutritional intake, getting enough food and vitamins to enhance survivability. **Sensory Specific Satiety was evolution's version of one-a-day multivitamins.**

Furthermore, by inducing satiety rapidly from one specific food, it would prevent ingesting too much of a food that might be a potential toxin. Consequently, the desire for that food would decrease after eating a specific amount before death could occur. Therefore, there is a strong evolutionary connection for Sensory Specific Satiety to enhance the survival of the human species.

Additional Findings

Sensory Specific Satiety has many implications and scientists are continuing to discover more and more. The following are some interesting additional findings:

1. Categories of Foods

The two major categories of sweet versus salty are somewhat divisive categories in Sensory Specific Satiety. To a certain degree, savory foods will have an impact on the satiety of other savory foods and sweet foods will have an impact on the satiety of other sweet foods but savory and sweet foods have far less impact on each other. That's why you would be able to eat ice cream (sweet) after feeling full from pizza (savory), but if you were offered potato chips or salty pretzels after feeling full from pizza, you would probably say no.

2. Volume of Food

Calories have far less of an impact than the volume of a specific food that you eat. For example, a piece of cake baked with a low caloric sweetener would have the same effect on satiety as the same size piece of cake laden with sugar that contained a higher caloric content.

3. Variety of Foods

The more variety of foods that are available at a given meal, the longer it will take for satiety to set in. In essence, more variety equals more potential calories consumed at any given meal. That's the reason that you tend to eat a larger amount of food and ingest a larger amount of calories at a buffet where an infinite number and types of foods are available, both savory and sweet. In addition, the time honored tradition of having appetizers before the meal begins encourages people to consume more calories because the shape, texture, and aroma of these additional foods can be far different than the ones consumed at the main meal.

4. Length of Sensory Specific Satiety

Sensory Specific Satiety can last twenty minutes or longer. This depends on the types of foods being eaten. Fatty foods tend to induce satiety for a shorter period of time whereas carbohydrates and fiber-rich foods tend to induce it for longer periods.

Short Term vs. Long Term Sensory Specific Satiety

The form of Sensory Specific Satiety that we have been speaking about is short term and is defined by individual foods consumed at a single meal. There is also a long-term version of Sensory Specific Satiety.[25] Long term Sensory Specific Satiety was discovered in a study of an Ethiopian refugee camp where it was found that refugees displayed a decreased appeal for their three normally-eaten foods over a period of six months as opposed to three other regular foods that they had not been eating. This finding was compared to new refugees who had not experienced any decrease in the pleasantness of the same meals after a shorter period of time. In this study, it was also determined that the decrease in the pleasantness of these foods directly corresponded to the intensity of the flavors. The higher the intensity, the higher the likelihood that long term Sensory Specific Satiety would arise. This type of satiety mainly deals with foods that comprise the major portion of the meal. For example, you would tend to lose your desire to eat meatloaf over time if it were given to you every night.

As you can see, Sensory Specific Satiety can be received as both positive and negative given the variety of foods that are available to us today. The more variety that we have, the more we tend to eat. In addition, our current food choices tend to be overly laden with unnecessary calories as compared to the size of the portions. Ounce per ounce, foods today have a much higher caloric intake than they have had in the past. Add to this people's continual cravings for "new" varieties of foods and you have a formula for disaster—more and more calories available at every meal. I can remember when granola was first introduced years ago. It was advertised as a very healthy choice made with natural grains. Today, you would hardly recognize it if you compared it to the original variety. There are so many variations of granola and each one contains more calories than the last.

Sensory Specific Satiety and Obesity

If you are one of the millions of people who are obese, you are probably wondering why the natural process of Sensory Specific Satiety doesn't seem to work for you. Sensory Specific Satiety works on an individual basis. The point of satiety for a specific food for you will probably be different than the satiety point for someone else.

There is also evidence to suggest that chronic overeaters have a reduced Sensory Specific Satiety reflex. In other words, this group can eat more before feeling full. One reason for this is that those who are obese have "super hedonics." To people who are obese, pleasant foods are super pleasant as compared to the non-obese. This was demonstrated by Dr. Linda Bartoshuk at Yale in a study of 4,299 subjects. She presented her findings of this investigation in 2006, stating that those who are obese are "living in an affectively more pleasant food world than do the non-obese." This suggests that when obese people enjoy food, they enjoy it much more than others, and when they love food, they have a much greater propensity to eat more of it than the non-obese who love the same food. People who are obese thus experience food differently than the non-obese. It is of a stronger and greater desire. There is almost an emotional attachment to the food.

Olfactory Sensory Specific Satiety

In a study conducted in 2005, it was demonstrated that Sensory Specific Satiety can be achieved just by chewing food the same amount of time as you normally would before swallowing it. In addition, it was also demonstrated in this study that the smelling of the foods for approximately the same amount of time as you would have chewed them induced olfactory Sensory Specific Satiety.[26] Both of these findings demonstrated that food does not have to enter the gastrointestinal system nor produce caloric intake into the body to induce Sensory Specific Satiety, and that the sense of smell could have a direct impact to the body's regulation of weight.

Chapter 7

THE ACCIDENTAL DISCOVERY OF THE SMELL-TASTE-WEIGHT CONNECTION

While I have worked for many years as a neurologist and psychiatrist, it is no secret by now that I am not a weight-loss specialist. However, the studies I have done and the patients I have treated for smell and taste related issues have led me to what I believe is an incredible breakthrough in the world of weight-loss. Let me briefly share the journey with you.

The Smell & Taste Treatment and Research Foundation in Chicago, which opened in 1987, is one of a handful of centers in the world devoted to the clinical treatment and research of smell and taste disorders. Our patients travel to us from all over the world. At the foundation, we see a wide spectrum of patients who have lost their sense of smell or taste, largely due to head trauma from a motor vehicle accident. Some patients have odor-induced symptoms, including exposure to smells that cause migraines or other headaches. Others complain of confusion, anxiety, dizziness and nausea, odor-induced panic disorders, odor-induced reactivation of post-traumatic stress disorders, or odor-induced seizure disorders. Patients also display hyperosmia, or an increased ability or sensitivity to smells. The list goes on and on.

The people we see in our office have been to an average of seven physicians before they come to us. What's more, they have often been misdiagnosed with a primary psychiatric disorder. Our evaluations show that their olfactory and gustatory (senses of smell and taste) complaints are quite real and due to a whole host of diverse medical and smell-taste dysfunctions.

Much of medicine is based on pattern recognition of symptoms. Medical knowledge shows us that when a patient presents a specific list of symptoms, we can diagnose the disease or disorder by comparing those same symptoms with known diseases or disorders.

I began to observe that patients with brain injuries from head trauma who lost their sense of smell had gained 10 to 20 pounds. As I previously mentioned, 90% of what we call taste is actually smell, so the patients who had lost their sense of smell had also lost the ability to taste foods. You would normally think that if they lost their ability to taste, then they would probably lose weight since foods would become far less appealing to them, causing them to eat less. However, these patients were gaining weight. This sparked my interest since it seemed that the decrease in smell, taste and overall pleasantness of foods had a direct correlation with weight gain. My "ah-ha" moment arrived when I started to think about the possibilities of the opposite being true. If somehow, I could interact with, influence, or enhance the pleasantness of foods in people with a normal sense of smell, would they lose weight as well?

In the last chapter, you learned a number of things regarding Sensory Specific Satiety, including how the aroma of food could induce this state on its own. I started to form a theory in my mind that the aromas of food could have a direct correlation to the amount of food that the body perceived as eaten. If somehow I could enhance or influence the aromas, could I make the body think that it has eaten more than it has and thus induce Sensory Specific Satiety at an earlier time and with less food? Based on this, I began to conduct a series of experiments.

In the first study, I wanted to confirm that specific aromas could directly influence satiety. In a double-blind study (neither the individuals nor the researchers knew who belonged to the control group and the experimental group), we placed specific aromas in plastic test tubes and asked 104 subjects to remove the top and sniff the test tubes three times in each nostril whenever they felt like eating. Each participant received two weeks of an active odorant versus two weeks of a placebo. (A placebo is a substance with no pharmacological effect but is administered as a control in testing a biologically active preparation.) After two weeks, those using the active odorant had an average weight loss of 1½ pounds. Although this suggested that odors might potentially help people lose weight, I remained skeptical because the study lasted just two weeks. With this short duration, a roller coaster effect could occur of lost and gained weight if the participants stopped using the odorants.

Our next study included 3,193 people and was conducted over a six-month period. The subjects were instructed to inhale a specific odorant three times in each nostril whenever they felt like eating. Astonishingly, at the end of the six months, there was an average weight loss of 30 pounds per person or approximately five pounds per month (approximately 2% per month in average body weight).

I then presented the data ("Inhalation of Odorants for Weight Reduction") at the International Congress on Obesity meeting in 1994, explaining the possible reasons for weight loss using this methodology along with some of the difficulties we encountered with this study. Our hypothesis for this study was based on the theory that the potential reason for weight loss was due to the fact that olfactory aspects of eating play a far greater degree in inducing Sensory Specific Satiety then was previously believed. The olfactory bulb at the top of the nose has the primary function of transmitting smell information to the brain by sending signals to the hypothalamus, a portion of the brain where hunger is controlled. Perhaps the increased levels of odors stimulated the hypothalamus in such a way that it was as if the body already had eaten certain foods. In this way, the odors may have been logged into the food diary of the hypothalamus. This correlated with our findings that frequency of sniffing aromas was an indicator of the amount of weight loss. Subjects recorded inhaling between 19 and 288 sniffs per day, averaging one sniff every six minutes while awake. The more frequently the subjects sniffed, the more weight they lost, which indicated the body had interpreted these odorants as already having eaten the food.

There were also a number of other reasons that could have induced the weight loss using this method. It could have been that the odorants reminded the people not to eat since this was a group of people who were more motivated to lose weight. Under this construct, the more motivated they were, the more they would use the method, i.e., sniffing. We know that motivation and compliance are the main factors in the reduction of addictive behaviors.

Alternatively, the odors could have acted as a distraction mechanism. Instead of grabbing a donut, the subjects grabbed the odorants. Not only did they have a physical action to replace eating, but their routine behavior of eating was replaced by a different cognitive behavior, sniffing. The odors induced weight loss with a smell-taste trigger that allowed participants to "read their own fuel-gauge" and see if their bodies were energy empty and required refueling. In this way, the odors may have acted as an external source to induce self-monitoring.

In addition, the odors may have acted to induce weight loss by inhibiting the well-known Pavlovian-conditioned response. With this reflex, when you smell a food, it induces hunger and you eat the food. By sniffing the odorants independent of food, this reflex may have been reversed so that when actual foods were presented with actual food odors, there was less of a response, and therefore, less of a demand to eat the food. We theorized all of the above possibilities.

In designing the protocol for this study, we examined the aspects of using pleasant versus unpleasant odors. At first, we thought that an unpleasant odor would inhibit ingestion because, logically, if you smell something bad, you don't feel like eating anything and you may become nauseous. We found just the opposite. If people disliked the smell, they gained weight. They would use the odorant once, realize they hated it, and never use it again—ultimately leading to an alternative like food. If participants in the study liked the smell, the more they used it and the more weight they lost.

After our presentation at the meeting, we became aware that using odorants doesn't make for a very good physiologic method. Who wants to be seen sniffing vials at dinner parties and in restaurants? We're used to eating rather than sniffing our food. Also, some participants didn't follow our instructions and often stuck the aroma inhalers too far into their nostrils. Believe it or not, the police called occasionally asking for explanations of what these people were sniffing. This convinced us that the odorants may not be the best vehicle for developing a proper, long-term approach to achieving permanent weight loss.

Based on this, we wanted to start experimenting with actual food rather than using something as a potential substitute for eating. We didn't want to develop specific foods from scratch, but rather we wanted to test something that could be added to foods to speed up Sensory Specific Satiety. We concluded that the most efficient method of achieving this would be to develop some type of food additive that you could sprinkle on all foods, which would interact with and intensify the taste of foods and make the body perceive that it had eaten more than it had, reducing calories and thus achieving weight loss.

We first went back and examined the research on Sensory Specific Satiety that determined that salty foods had an effect on inducing satiety on other salty foods and sweet foods had the same effect on other sweet foods. Based on this research, we developed two specific types of food sprinkles—one that would be used on salty foods and another that would be used on sweet foods. We called these sprinkles, "Tastants." We began testing various formulations for these Tastants over a period of years. **After testing over 4,000 different Tastant formulations, we finalized six "salty" flavors and six "sweet" flavors that had the maximum impact in inducing Sensory Specific Satiety and weight loss in individual subjects.** Even though the Tastants were to be used on salty and sweet foods, they did not contain any salt or sugar.

We conducted an initial pilot study with 92 subjects over a six month period in 2002. Participants were asked to sprinkle these Tastants on their foods whenever they ate—the savory ones on foods typically seasoned with salt (meats, vegetables, pasta, etc.), and the sweet ones on sweeter foods (cakes, fruits, etc.). Using these Tastants resulted in substantial weight loss. Compared to a control group that used no Tastants, those who used Tastants lost an average of 34 pounds over a six-month period (approximately 2.1% body mass per month)! The greatest results were seen in those participants with the normal ability to smell and taste.

In 2004, I wanted to test this process on a much larger population base. In this next clinical trial, 1,436 people finished the study. A non-treatment control group of 100 individuals were randomly selected to not use the Tastants. Both groups were instructed not to change their eating or exercise routines over the course of the study. Weight and body mass index (BMI) were measured for both groups before and after the study. **The test group using the Tastants experienced an average weight loss of 30.5 pounds, and an average BMI decrease of 5 points, over a period of six months.** The control group who used nothing lost an average of only 2 pounds, with an average BMI decrease of 0.3 points over the same period.

Word spread quickly about the study and this unusual method of approaching weight loss. *Dateline NBC* wanted to do an exposé that would disprove the efficacy of this weight-loss method. At a restaurant in Texas, *Dateline NBC* had the cameras rolling while a dozen people who had participated in Dr. Hirsch's study sat down for a meal. These same people kept a video diary of themselves using the Tastants for six months on a consistent basis. The videos were provided to *Dateline NBC*. To their surprise, all of the people lost a substantial amount of weight.

Prior to the *Dateline NBC* story, my mission was purely research and I hadn't considered the idea of making the Tastants available to the public. But soon I realized the impact that this research could have on changing and improving many lives. While the public interest grew and the plans to make the product available were set in place, my research did not feel complete.

Most recently, and most notable is the independent double-blind placebo controlled study. The one aspect that we wanted to specifically test was the act of sprinkling something on the food. An act, such as this, could make someone more cognizant of what they are eating and thus stimulate them to eat less and/or lower calorie foods. In order to eliminate the act of sprinkling as a cause of weight loss, we consulted an independent, third-party laboratory. In this study both groups received Tastants to use, but only the active group was given the Sensa Tastants. The other group was given a placebo form of Tastants without our specifically designed formulation.

Participants using the active Tastants experienced an average weight loss of 27.5 pounds in six months. Participants in the placebo group actually gained an average of nearly one-half pound in the same time period. The results of this study are significant because they provide further support for the results obtained in my 2004 study where participants experienced an average weight loss of 30.5 pounds in six months. No longer could we consider the possibility that the mere act of sprinkling something on food was making people more cognizant of what or how much they were eating, thus causing people to put their fork down. This last study proved conclusively that the weight loss was caused specifically by the individual formulations of the active Tastants.

I probably would have laughed if someone told me 25 years ago that as a neurologist and psychiatrist, I would also be the creator of a weight-loss program. I share this story of discovery with you so that you too can understand how a doctor who specializes in the treatment of smell and taste would become the doctor who would help you overcome your weight struggles. Having seen the results of the Tastants, I am excited to share them with you. As a doctor who cares for the well-being of his patients, I have developed the Sensa Weight-Loss Program, a 3–Level program that will not only help you lose weight, but also give you the tools to live a healthier lifestyle and begin your healthy relationship with food.

PART II

THE SENSA WEIGHT-LOSS PROGRAM

Chapter 8

LEVEL 1
THE SENSA TASTANT SYSTEM

Understanding the method behind the Sensa Weight-Loss Program is the first step to achieving a thinner, healthier you. You have learned how smell and taste play an active role in our daily lives and how these two senses can affect everything from our memories to our appetite. You now know how my accidental discovery led to the development of the Sensa Tastants. Now, you can begin to use the Tastants to help you eat less.

What are Sensa Tastants?

Though Tastants may sound like magic fairy dust, the ingredients in Sensa can be found in foods that you eat everyday. The definition of a tastant is any substance that is capable of eliciting gustatory excitation.[27] Sounds complex—but all that means is "something that stimulates your sense of taste," and as you know now, taste and

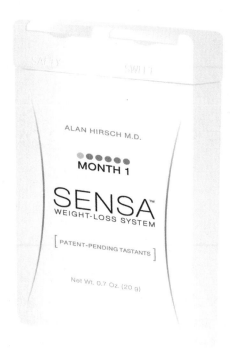

Figure 2: Sensa Tastant Shaker—Month 1

smell are very closely connected. **Sensa Tastants are sodium-free, sugar-free, calorie free and gluten-free, and there are no stimulants, drugs or MSG. If you have specific dietary concerns, no flavors are derived from meat sources and there is no mushroom, nutmeg, cinnamon, fish, or garlic. Some flavors may contain milk and soy derived ingredients, but in very small traces.**

The Sensa Tastants are a proprietary and patent-pending blend of different tastes and flavors that I found encourage satiety, making people eat less and lose weight. As I discussed before, I tested over 4,000 different combinations before I solidified the final 12 that make up Sensa. While many of the Tastants I tested encouraged people to eat more, I concluded my study with a final number of 12 (six sweet and six salty) that, when used in a certain progression, achieved the maximum amount of weight loss.

How to Use

The Sensa Tastants are organized into a six-month system—two shakers for each month. The two shakers make up a 30–day supply of Tastants so that at the end of each month your shakers should be empty and you will be ready to move onto the next month. We created the two sets with ease in mind. This way, you can keep one at home and keep another one with you when you're eating outside of your home. You should sprinkle Sensa Tastants liberally on everything you eat—whether it's a full meal or a snack in between. You should use Sensa Tastants on all solid and semi-solid foods. The only items you don't need to sprinkle Sensa Tastants on are liquids such as drinks, soups, etc. I found that the Tastants weren't formulated specifically for liquids because they would sink to the bottom or float without engaging the senses. Semi-solids like hearty soups, stews, and cereal are OK.

When I was developing the Sensa Tastants, I found that certain blends of scents and flavors showed the greatest affect on weight loss—but only when used in 30–day increments. Because our

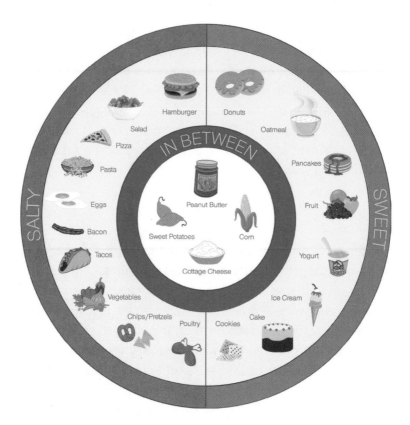

Figure 3: Checklist of Salty vs. Sweet Usage

bodies can adjust to scents, it is important to start the new set of Tastants every 30 days—even if you find you have some left over. It's important to keep your olfactory senses stimulated with the different scents and tastes to achieve maximum results. If your senses get bored, the Tastants won't have the necessary effect.

Each month is comprised of a unique and proprietary blend of "salty" and "sweet" Tastants. While you won't notice much of a change in the taste of your food (if you even notice a change at all), the "salty" and "sweet" were created to help you determine which foods to use the Tastants on. Fruit, baked goods, and ice cream are considered sweet. Eggs, most meats and chips are considered salty. There are some in between foods that get some people confused, such as cottage cheese, corn, and potatoes, but what I always tell my patients is that you can't make a mistake! If you like fruit in your cottage cheese, sweet might be your best choice. If you like your corn on the salty side, use the salty Tastants. If you really aren't sure, I recommend using the sweet Tastants. As long as you sprinkle Tastants on every thing you eat, you are using Sensa correctly.

Refer to Figure 3 for a list of typical foods that you would normally eat to demonstrate what type foods you would use the "salty" Tastants versus the "sweet" Tastants on.

Frequently Asked Questions

Some of the best questions and feedback we have received has been from Sensa users. I want to share some of the most frequently asked questions and answers with you so you too can find success with Sensa.

Where can I purchase the Sensa Tastants?

The Sensa Tastants are available as part of the Sensa Weight-Loss System. Please visit www.trysensa.com to order.

How do the Sensa Tastants work to help me lose weight?

Sensa Tastants were designed to induce Sensory Specific Satiety by working with the body's natural appetite suppressing system. Figure 4 illustrates how Sensory Specific Satiety works. For more information, use the DVD included in the book, which provides an explanation of the process.

THE SATIETY PROCESS:

HOW YOUR BODY KNOWS WHEN TO STOP EATING

1. Scents from foods cause nerve receptors in the nose to send signals to the olfactory bulb.

2. When the olfactory bulb is stimulated, it triggers the satiety center in the hypothalamus.

3. This triggers the release of hormones that suppress hunger and appetite.

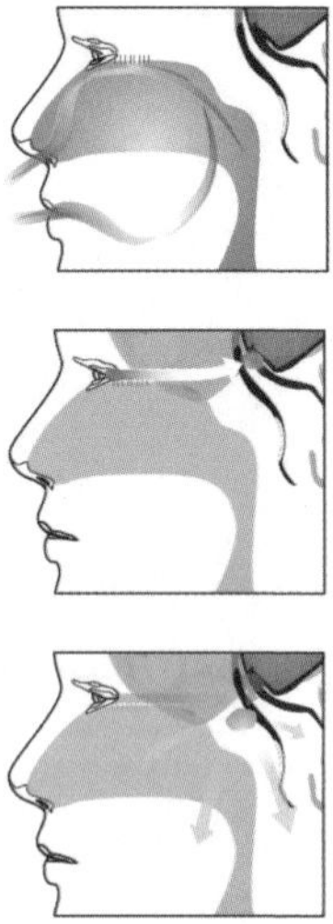

Figure 4: Sensory Specific Satiety: How Your Body Knows When to Stop Eating

What if I run out early?

If you run out early do not be alarmed, simply move on to the next month of Tastants. The two sets of Tastants per month should last you approximately 30 days, so if you finish ahead of schedule, you may want to try using the Tastants a bit more sparingly next month.

Do I discard the excess Tastants at the end of the month or finish them?

Both shakers for each month were designed as a 30–day supply. We recommend discarding the leftover Tastants as you need to move on to the next month's shakers for maximum results.

How much do I sprinkle exactly?

Sprinkle Sensa Tastants evenly on the entire surface of your food. The amount of Sensa Tastants depends on how large your meal is, so just use your best judgment and don't over think it. Please refer to Figure 5 for an example of how to sprinkle.

Do I sprinkle before or after cooking?

The Sensa Tastants should not be used before or while cooking your food. Sensa Tastants work best when you sprinkle it right before eating. This way, your sense of smell can properly interact with the Tastants.

Too Little

Just Right

Too Much

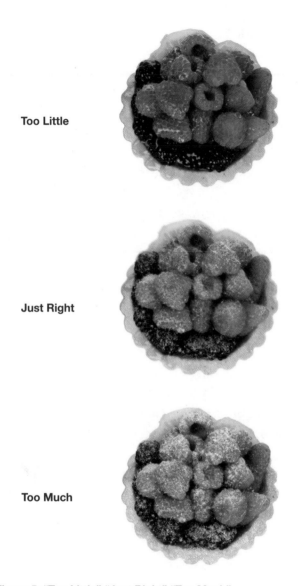

Figure 5: "Too Little" "Just Right" "Too Much"

Can I sprinkle my food when I am packing my lunch or do I have to do it just before eating?

I recommend sprinkling Sensa Tastants on your food right before you eat to achieve maximum results.

What happens at month seven?

If you wish to continue with the program past month six, you should start the system over with month one.

Do I need to put more Sensa Tastants on leftovers if I already put it on the first time?

To ensure that your sense of smell is properly engaged, I recommend you re-sprinkle leftovers with a second round of Sensa Tastants.

How do I get it to stick to foods like grapes, nuts or pretzels?

Some users have found that spraying a fine mist of water on grapes or strawberries to get the Sensa Tastants to stick is effective. You can also sprinkle Sensa Tastants over the plate or in the bag (chips or pretzels) so that the Tastants touch all of your food.

If I eat something like pasta or salad, do I have to re-sprinkle Sensa Tastants when I have eaten the top layer?

As long as you sprinkle Sensa Tastants over the entire surface of your meal, there is no need to re-sprinkle each layer.

How do you use Sensa Tastants in soup or smoothies?

You do not need to use Sensa Tastants in soup or smoothies, only on solid or semi-solid foods. You should use Sensa Tastants on cereals, chili or a hearty soup that has meat, vegetables or noodles.

Is it possible to sprinkle too much of the Sensa Tastants?

If you are finding that you are running out of Sensa Tastants long before the month is over, you may be using too much. There is no need to worry if you have used too much Sensa, just think about using less the next time.

Do you use Sensa Tastants on things like hard candy?

Yes, you should use Sensa Tastants on everything you eat for best results.

How should I store my Sensa Tastants?

Sensa Tastants should be stored in a cool, dry place. For best results, once opened, Sensa Tastants should be used within 30 days.

I have gained weight. What's going on?

Sensa Tastants are non-caloric and alone would not produce weight gain. The most likely reason that someone would gain weight when they begin Sensa is that they are not yet in tune with their body's hunger signals. Eat slowly, and pay attention. As soon as you START to feel full you should stop eating. Also, if you are already on another weight-loss program or diet at the time that you start Sensa, you should continue on that program and use Sensa in addition to it.

I'm eating more often. What's up?

Everyone reacts to the Tastants differently. Even though you are eating more often, you are probably still consuming less calories overall. In fact, having smaller, more frequent meals throughout the day is a highly effective way to boost your metabolism.

How long will it take until I lose weight?

There is no "typical" timeline for losing weight with Sensa. Although many people lose weight in the very first month, everyone experiences weight loss differently. Stick with the system and you will lose weight.

What if I am still eating my entire meal?

It is completely normal to eat your entire meal with Sensa Tastants. However, since you are trying to lose weight, it is important that you stop eating when your body signals "satiety" or "fullness." You should stop at the onset of these signals, not once you are already feeling full.

What if I still feel hungry?

Go ahead and eat. Just be sure to use Sensa Tastants on every single meal and snack, from your morning cereal, to salads, chocolate chip cookies, and potato chips. *Consistency is the key.*

What long-term results can I expect?

Many study participants reported continued weight loss. We believe this may be because the body gradually adjusts over time to smaller portions, making it easier to practice moderation. Exercise and healthy eating are also encouraged to achieve long-term sustainable weight loss.

Can I use Sensa if I want to lose less than 30 pounds?
Sensa is effective for anyone who wants to lose weight, regardless of the amount.

What exactly is in Sensa Tastants?
Sensa Tastants contains maltodextrin (derived from corn from the USA), tricalcium phosphate, silica, and natural and artificial flavors. Sensa Tastants also contains soy and milk ingredients. Sensa Tastants are sodium-free, sugar-free, calorie free, gluten-free, and there are no stimulants, drugs, or MSG.

What are the natural and artificial flavorings?
The exact combinations of the Sensa Tastants blends are proprietary and patent-pending. However, no flavors are derived from meat sources and there is no mushroom, nutmeg, cinnamon, fish or garlic.

Is there soy and milk in the product?
Soy and milk ingredients may be found as constituents of some of the natural and artificial flavoring agents. The soy in Sensa Tastants is soy-lecithin.

What is maltodextrin?
The maltodextrin in Sensa Tastants is made up of easily digestible carbohydrates made from natural corn starch.

Is it FDA approved?

As a food product, FDA approval is not required for Sensa. All of Sensa's ingredients are on the FDA designation list of GRAS — Generally Recognized as Safe.

Is this a vegan product?

Some flavors may contain milk ingredients.

Are there side effects or negatives to using Sensa Tastants?

Sensa Tastants work solely on smell and taste, and all ingredients are GRAS, or generally recognized as safe, by the FDA. Sensa's ingredients can be found in common foods such as baby food, yogurt, pudding, or salad dressing. Sensa does contain soy and milk ingredients. Please consult with your physician if you have any food sensitivities or allergies. If you experience any unusual side effects, please consult your physician or stop using the product.

How old do I have to be to use Sensa Tastants?

Sensa has been studied on adults only, so there is no data available about its effectiveness in helping children lose weight. As a result, we do not recommend our products for use by children.

Can I use Sensa Tastants if I am breastfeeding, have diabetes, high blood pressure, or any other medical condition or concern?

While the ingredients found in Sensa Tastants are safe, we recommend that you consult your physician before using Sensa Tastants or starting any weight-loss plan if you have any medical concerns whatsoever.

What if I have completely lost my sense of taste and smell? Will this work for me?

Unfortunately, Sensa Tastants will not be effective if you have no sense of taste or smell, and may be less effective for those with diminished sense of taste or smell.

Tips for Sucess

Remembering to use Sensa Tastants on everything you eat should be the most challenging part of this program (and I think it's safe to say that this isn't particularly difficult). Whether it's leaving a note on your refrigerator or tying a string on your wrist, Sensa will become second nature to you as you sprinkle at every meal. Many Sensa users have formed Sensa Support Groups. They check in with each other regularly keeping their fellow Sensa users motivated and sprinkling. Finding a system that works for you will make this simple program even easier.

While the beauty of Sensa is that you can still enjoy the foods you love while losing weight, you must always remember that the key to weight loss is consuming less and moving more. The point is that you can still do this without feeling like you have to completely change your lifestyle, count calories, order packaged meals, or hit the gym for hours a day. The Sensa Tastants are the first part to this simple and unique weight-loss journey. You will start to see and *enjoy* the smaller portions that make you feel full. You will start to lose the weight that has prevented you from being physically active.

While I hope my explanation of the Tastants and the science behind them has given you a greater understanding of the program, I know that the most inspiring aspect are the stories of real people who found success with Sensa and I am excited to share their journeys with you.

Chapter 9

SENSA SUCCESS STORIES

I am happy to share with you some of the real-life success stories from people who have benefited from The Sensa Tastant System. It is my hope that these participants in the program will inspire you and other readers to be brave and steadfast on your weight loss journey.

The following are wonderful stories from different users who have experienced personal success with Sensa. Individual results will vary as with any weight-loss program. Many of these results are not typical.

Gaylene

Lost 53 pounds

I am a 55 year old female who has always been in pretty good shape. I am 5'6" and currently weigh 136. After menopause the pounds just gradually kept creeping up to a whopping 187 pounds. Even though I eat pretty healthy, I found that they just kept creeping. I enjoy having a glass of wine most nights and I just did not want to give up my life style. Life is too short.

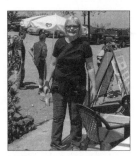

before

Enter Sensa—I started using Sensa and the first month noticed that I felt fuller faster, so I didn't eat as much. I lost about 4 pounds that first month. When I started month two (a new shaker), I did not notice the full feeling and was a little disappointed but kept sprinkling anyway. I lost a few more pounds.

Although I kept sprinkling for months three and four, I did not notice anything but I did lose a few more pounds. I was questioning whether this stuff REALLY worked but I kept sprinkling. By months 5 and 6, the pounds just started melting away. It was unbelievable. My pants were

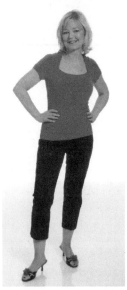

after

Results not typical. Individual results may vary.

fitting looser and looser and I lost that muffin bulge at my waist that I have had for so long.

Now I am 4 pant sizes smaller, healthier and happier . . . I am thrilled to say that SENSA IS GREAT. I had always planned to start exercising again (and still have not). I keep telling myself I have a pretty active life with 4 dogs and 2 kids, so I do keep busy. I do not have the time to plan all my meals, eat only certain foods, take pills, or exercise. But I do have time to sprinkle, which is what I do. I am soooo happy I did and hope to lose just a couple more pounds. Everyone is amazed, I look like I did in high school. Also, I enjoy eating healthy, but will always have an occasional slice of pizza with my kids and a glass of wine at night.

I look and feel great. I hope to never be that heavy again. Now I have so many people trying sensa because of how it worked for me. I would recommend it to anyone as long as they have the discipline to just keep sprinkling.

Deanna E.   *Lost 45 pounds in six months*

I have a 3 year old and a 6 year old. I gained 30 to 40 pounds with each baby and the weight just didn't come off. I tried to lose weight with all the other advertised diet programs in the marketplace. I lost a little bit of weight but then as soon as I stopped the diets, I gained all the weight back and sometimes more! I actually went from a size 18 to a size 10 and lost 45 pounds using Sensa.

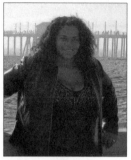

before

*I went to the mall the other day and I passed Lane Bryant. I started to go in and I realized I'm just not that person anymore. And it felt wonderful. **I got my sexy back and my husband won't stop chasing me around the house.***

I'm a changed person.

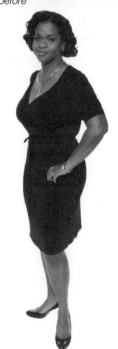

after

Results not typical. Individual results may vary.

94

Martha O.

Lost 35 pounds

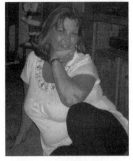

before

I had been slender for a lot of my young adult life. I never worried about food or my weight. I'm originally from South America and in my early 20s went through a very rough patch . . . I struggled through a divorce, and then left for the U.S. I felt isolated and turned to food for comfort. At that point, I gained 100 pounds in just about six months. Since then, I've been a yo-yo dieter.

The biggest misconception about being overweight is that people aren't trying to eat healthy or exercise. I like going for walks, I like eating healthy, but I also want to eat some of my favorite foods. The word "diet" gives me a headache. I have tried so many different diets, and I know that I haven't been successful with them because I always felt deprived.

When I first started using Sensa, I noticed a difference the first week in my eating habits, but I noticed the weight loss in the third week. Once I saw the results,

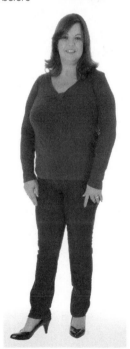

after

Results not typical. Individual results may vary.

it motivated me to start walking and eating healthier, but if I want a donut or chips, I can still have them. I have more energy now, I feel good about the weight I have lost and am confident that I'll reach my goals with this program. **It has been the easiest thing I've tried. It's like my body finally has the internal portion control I've been missing.**

I now have a beautiful 13–year-old daughter and the best thing my daughter says to me is, "Mom, you're not having those side effects where you're in a terrible mood or you have a headache all the time or your arms are cramping, And you're not complaining."

That's what diets usually do to me. My daughter is now so proud of me. She sees the portions I eat and gets a sense of healthy portions for herself and what it means to eat in moderation.

George S.

Lost 25 pounds

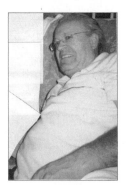

before

I'm 55, and I have a five-year-old daughter. For me, the best part of losing weight was the effect on our relationship, being able to jump and run and play with her. Before, I was hesitant because I felt pain and didn't have energy. Now she says "I love you, Daddy" five or six times a day!

People call me grandpa all the time. Now I say, "You think I'm a grandpa? Let's run from here to there and see who's grandpa. Try me out." I couldn't have said that six months ago. Twenty-five pounds is too much extra weight to carry around. Now that it's gone, what a difference. **It's changed my life tremendously. I feel energized.**

You hear about different products, and they just don't work. I tried a few other diets, and they just didn't work for me. I was never satisfied, and felt like I was always going back to bad eating habits.

With Sensa, I felt like it became part of my daily routine some time after about three weeks or a month and my appetite was just not there anymore. I felt full. What I really liked was that there was no taste, and it was very easy to apply.

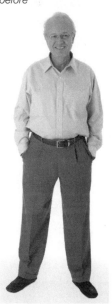

after

Results not typical. Individual results may vary.

Josh Z.

Lost 53 pounds in nine months

I'm 35 and have tried every diet available. I was ready for a change in my life. I was tired of being the fat guy at the beach who didn't want to take his shirt off or the person at the swim party that didn't want to jump in the pool. With Sensa, I've learned that portion control is very important. I've started to feel aware of what I'm eating and notice that my cravings have subsided. When I sprinkle it on the food, it gives me the opportunity to be aware of what I'm doing.

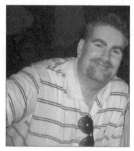

before

My whole life has been up and down with the dieting. Usually I don't really last on diets . . . two to four months. I'm at six months with Sensa and I use it every single day. It really has become an integral part of my life.

Since using Sensa, all my friends have commented that I look really great. I went from a size 46 down to a size 40 and took six inches off my waist in six months using Sensa. I can fit into skinnier jeans now, which is important to me.

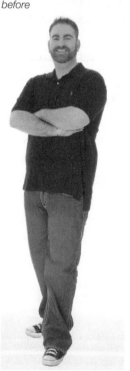

after

Results not typical. Individual results may vary.

When I started going out for sushi, I would have a $100 to $120 sushi bill. **Now that I sprinkle the Sensa on my dinners, I'm full at half the price and I'm not sacrificing eating great food. It's just a reduction in food. It has not only changed my appearance, but helped me keep more money in my wallet.**

It's almost second nature. It's extremely easy to use. The main thing is you have to carry it with you and you have to use it. All you do is take it out, and whatever food you are eating, salty or sweet, go to that side of the container, sprinkle the Sensa on, and eat away. There's no change in texture or taste. Everything tastes the same. In time, you'll notice your appetite is decreasing but you're not sacrificing what you're eating.

I feel great now that I've lost the weight. I'm able to do a lot more things. I'm not snoring at night and I think my sleep apnea has gone down. I'd like to lose another 40 pounds and I'm confident that if I stick with Sensa, I will attain that goal.

Dina C.

Lost 37 pounds in eight months

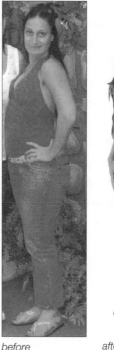

before   after

I'm a 29–year-old third grade teacher, so I need to keep my energy up. I tried a diet where you drink two shakes and "one sensible meal a day." That just didn't cut it for me. I was starving.

I saw my friend who was literally shrinking, and asked her what she was doing. When she told me that she was putting sprinkles on her food and they made her eat less, I thought she was joking. But then she showed me Sensa and I decided to try it.

I didn't see results right away, but since Sensa worked for my friend, I kept using it and didn't give up. By the end of the second week, I started to see a little difference. Then, after the fourth week, my weight loss really became evident.

I love my food and don't want to give it up. I have a big family; we are always at each other's houses surrounded by good food. With Sensa, I can still eat all that food, but I just don't eat as much of it.

Results not typical. Individual results may vary.

Adriana J.   *Lost 12 pounds in one month*

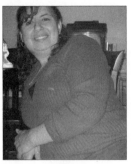

When my cousin told me about Sensa, I thought, "Okay, I've tried everything under the sun. I'll give this a try too."

The first thing I noticed was how good my food tasted. Sensa didn't change the taste of my food. Then I noticed that I wasn't eating everything on my plate. It took about a month to really kick in.

before

We women want instant results, when it comes to weight loss. I had to be patient and just kept using it at every meal. I soon noticed that I wasn't eating as much and losing weight. I remember thinking, "It's working—it's actually working!" When I saw the results I was motivated to start working out and walking more. I actually bought a bike and now ride with my son every night.

The weight has come off gradually, which I think is better than trying to get a quick fix. It's healthier and it's easier to keep the weight off than with crash diets, where your metabolism goes crazy and you gain all the weight back.

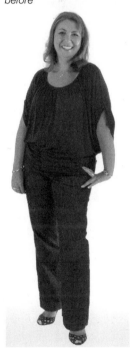

after

Results not typical. Individual results may vary.

I try to eat healthy, but one thing I always hated about diets was going to work and staring at the birthday cake or donuts everyone else was eating and not being able to eat any. **With Sensa, I don't worry about what I'm eating. I don't have any restrictions. I don't weigh in at meetings. I don't count anything. I can cook what I like, sprinkle on Sensa, and just don't eat as much.**

Jessica L.

Lost 34 pounds in six months

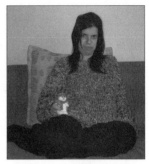

When I moved to Los Angeles, I put on a lot of weight. As a makeup artist, I have lots of friends who are models, and they were always getting me to try new diet pills. I just felt hungry all the time and became discouraged because I wasn't losing any weight.

before

With Sensa, it took about a month to see a real difference. I stuck with it and the pounds just started coming off. I couldn't believe how easy it was.

I have lots of early call times—5 or 6 a.m.—and I'm usually on the set until midnight, so I don't have time to go to the gym. I bring Sensa with me to shoots and it keeps me from over-eating.

My favorite thing about losing weight has been buying new clothes! It's fun to try on nice clothes and have them fit.

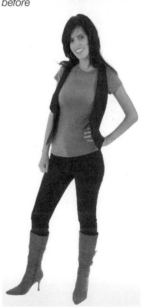

after

Results not typical. Individual results may vary.

Michelle F.

Lost 40 pounds in 6 months

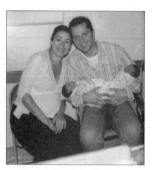

before

I never really had a weight problem until I had my twins. I gained almost 60 pounds with my pregnancy and had about 40 pounds left to lose. My body just didn't bounce back as easily as it did after my first pregnancy. It was difficult to lose the baby weight, because I was so busy with my twins and my toddler. There was no time to count calories or workout.

*A friend of mine told me about Sensa, and I thought, "This sounds too good to be true. This is way too easy," but my friend was successful on the program, so I thought I'd give it a try. **And by the end of the six months, I had lost all of my pregnancy weight!***

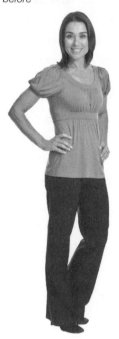

after

Results not typical. Individual results may vary.

Chapter 10

LEVEL 2
THE SENSA
SATIETY SYSTEM

We have just left Level 1 of the Sensa Weight-Loss Program—
the Sensa Tastant System. This is by far the easiest, simplest way
to lose weight and also is the best way to kick-start yourself to a
healthier lifestyle. My experience has shown that dieting is a no win
situation. It is neither desirable nor sustainable for a long period of
time. People give up quickly and gravitate back to their own individual comfort zone, eating the foods they love and exercising very
little. With Level 1, there is no change to your present lifestyle. You
are free to enjoy all of your favorite foods and still lose weight. There
is no pain or deprivation whatsoever. The Sensa Tastant System is
like the "missing link" of weight loss programs. The problem with
traditional programs is that they induce lots of pain before any real
pleasure is felt. Sensa is different because it induces pleasure without pain. The pleasure that you receive from losing weight without

pain of deprivation and restriction is the essence to the success of the program. There is no other program like it.

As people start to lose weight, they become motivated. This motivation takes the form of wanting to do additional things to become more successful and increase their speed of weight loss toward achieving their ultimate ideal weight goal. This motivation also takes the form of wanting to live a healthier lifestyle as they find themselves being able to do things that they couldn't before, like touching their toes, walking without losing their breath and having more energy. All of these things are the positive consequences of losing weight. That's why I have designed two additional levels so that you can advance your pace and eventually graduate to a healthier lifestyle. The 3 level program acts like a domino effect—the more successful you are, the more successful you want to become. The program is customizable. If and when you are ready, Level 2—the Sensa Satiety System, awaits you. Again this system is a simple, easy, and lifestyle-friendly approach to fast tracking your weight loss to reach your individual goals.

The Level 2 is a two-part, graduated system. The first step shows you how you can begin to make substitutions to incorporate higher satiety foods into your daily meals. The second features a whole list of high satiety recipes that you can pick and choose from and lays out a complete two week program that you can follow as you feel additional motivation.

Step 1
High Satiety Foods

The Level 1, Sensa Tastant System helps you to take in fewer calories; you feel satisfied with the same foods that you have always enjoyed while eating less of them. How do you go to the next level? How can you still enjoy your favorite foods but lose even more weight? The answer lies in something called the Satiety Index.

Let's look at an example of a person who is not presently on the Sensa Weight-Loss Program. Mary is hungry all the time. She wakes up each morning and before going to work fixes herself a traditional breakfast of bacon, eggs, and coffee. At mid-morning, she's practically starving. She goes on break and gets some snacks from the company cafeteria—a banana and a soda. By noontime, she can't wait to go to lunch. She has a cheeseburger with all the trimmings and French fries. By 3 PM, she can't wait to take her break and hit the cafeteria again. She buys a candy bar and another soda. She doesn't feel like cooking a whole dinner so she picks up a foot-long submarine sandwich and another soda. Before bed, she indulges in a scoop of her favorite sorbet. At the end of the day, she looks back and wonders why she was so hungry all day long. Mary is currently 100 pounds over her ideal weight.

Mary begins the Sensa Weight-Loss Program with Level 1. She starts to use the Tastants and after two months, she has lost a total of ten pounds. She's still enjoying all her favorite foods but she finds that she is eating less of them. She can't finish all of her breakfast, she's cut her snacks in half in between meals and she can only eat half of the portion sizes at dinner that she normally eats. She's never experienced losing weight in such an easy manner. She is full, satisfied and dropping pounds. Life is good and Mary is motivated to go to the next level—the Sensa Satiety System.

Susanna Holt at the University of Sydney was the first researcher to index foods and categories of foods based on satiety. In her study, 38 foods with the same 240 calorie portion size were evaluated over a two-hour period to measure the degree of satiety as compared to that of white bread. **What was most notable in this study was that fatty, energy-dense foods served in the smallest amounts stimulated the desire to eat.** These foods promoted an over-consumption of energy and led to obesity. Foods such as fried chicken from your favorite restaurant would fall into this category. There is no secret that when eating fat-rich foods you consume more calories. And, since you have picked up this book, you are probably one of the millions of people who find it difficult to go "cold turkey" and stop eating fat-rich foods completely. That is exactly why the Sensa Tastant System has been so successful.

Let's get back to Mary. Mary probably ate almost 2,700 calories a day, before she started the Sensa Tastant System. With that level of calories, you would think that she would have felt "stuffed" all day but she didn't. Why? She filled her day with a menu of low satiety foods, foods that left her feeling hungry after a short period of time. After she went on the Sensa Tastant System, the amount of food that she consumed decreased along with a decrease in calories. But what if Mary understood the Satiety Index developed by Susanna Holt? Do you think Mary could have made some better choices at meals just by substituting some foods at her meal with others and in doing this consume even less calories? Absolutely!

The Satiety Index

Let's first take a look at the Satiety Index of foods.

Bakery Products	Overall Satiety	Group Satiety
Croissant	47%	1.0
Cake	65%	1.4
Doughnuts	68%	1.4
Cookies	120%	2.6
Crackers	127%	2.7

Carbohydrate-Rich Foods	Overall Satiety	Group Satiety
White bread	100%	1.0
French fries	116%	1.2
White pasta	119%	1.2
Brown rice	132%	1.3
White rice	138%	1.4
Grain bread	154%	1.5
Whole meal bread	157%	1.6
Brown pasta	188%	1.9
Potatoes, boiled	323%	3.2

Snacks and Confectionary	Overall Satiety	Group Satiety
Mars candy bar	70%	1.0
Peanuts	84%	1.2
Yogurt	88%	1.3
Crisps	91%	1.3

Ice cream	96%	1.4
Jellybeans	118%	1.7
Popcorn	154%	2.2

Breakfast Cereals with Milk	**Overall Satiety**	**Group Satiety**
Muesli	100%	1.0
Sustain	112%	1.1
Special K	116%	1.2
Cornflakes	118%	1.2
Honey Smacks	132%	1.3
All-Bran	151%	1.5
Porridge/Oatmeal	209%	2.1

Protein-Rich Foods	**Overall Satiety**	**Group Satiety**
Lentils	133%	1.0
Cheese	146%	1.1
Eggs	150%	1.1
Baked beans	168%	1.3
Beef	176%	1.3
Ling fish	225%	1.7

Fruits	**Overall Satiety**	**Group Satiety**
Bananas	118%	1.0
Grapes	162%	1.4
Apples	197%	1.7
Oranges	202%	1.7

You will notice that there are six foods groups—Bakery Products, Carbohydrate Rich Foods, Snacks and Confectionary, Breakfast Cereals with Milk, Protein-Rich Foods, and Fruits. The chart lists the foods in two ways. First, the "Overall Satiety," percentage rating compares all the foods on the chart as if they were grouped together. The percentage compares them to white bread, which equals 100%. As mentioned, this rating is for the same calorie amount in each food—240 calories. The higher the percentage, the higher the level of satiety the food produced as compared to the baseline food of white bread. For example, a 240–calorie portion of eggs (150%) produced 50% more satiety than a 240 portion of white bread, whereas, a croissant (47%) produced less than 50% the amount of satiety. This satiety level was measured over a two hour period so it was considered short term satiety. The second column, "Group Satiety," compares the level of satiety as compared to the individual food group listed. For example, in the food group of "Breakfast Cereals with Milk," 240 calories of oatmeal (2.1) produced more than two times the amount of satiety as opposed to the same calorie level of muesli (1.0), whereas, in the food group of "Carbohydrate-Rich Foods," 240 calories of boiled potatoes (3.2) produced more than three times the amount of satiety as the same calorie level of white bread (1.0).

There were a few other things that Holt discovered. Fatty foods were not as satiating as people thought them to be. The reason could be that these foods may be recognized by the body as a group that should be stored for future use in emergencies. **Because the body doesn't recognize the fat as energy for immediate use, it doesn't tell the brain to cut hunger signals, so you go**

on wanting more. Carbohydrates are the opposite of fats. They raise blood glucose so the body knows it has gotten enough fuel, thus sending signals to say "we have received enough."

In our above example, if Mary began to have oatmeal for just one breakfast a week instead of her bacon and egg breakfast, she would begin to gain benefits from Level 2. This small change can result in her eating less during lunch that day because oatmeal will make her feel full for a longer period of time and she may also find herself cutting out her mid-morning snack. She can eventually graduate to eating oatmeal two to three times a week and additional pounds will come off even more quickly. If she would have chosen an orange instead of a banana during her midday snack, she may have felt less hungry at dinner and bypassed that sorbet for dessert. The point is that by starting to incorporate higher satiety foods into your menu while using the Sensa Tastants, you are taking the right steps to maximize your weight loss.

The Sensa Satiety System is a gradual process. I am not suggesting to completely change your entire eating habits. Becoming better educated about how foods interact with our bodies in making us feel satisfied will go a long way in helping us lose additional weight and become healthier.

In addition to adding more high-satiety foods to your diet, try these two simple tips in the first few weeks on Level 2.

1. Slow down while eating

The longer it takes you to finish a meal, the less you will eat overall. The less you eat the more weight you lose.

2. Eat foods that require more of an effort to consume.

For example, hot soups and stews that need to cool off between bites are better choices than cold salads. Foods with high liquid content such as soups and fruits tend to have a higher satiety level and possibly a lower calorie level as well. Whole oranges and apples and lightly steamed vegetables require more peeling and cutting than orange juice, applesauce, and purees. Spaghetti, which requires twirling it around a fork between bites, takes longer to eat than tortellini. Shrimp in their shells are a better choice than those that are already peeled.

The point of this program is to make losing weight simple and easy and to limit the amount of change you have to make to your daily routine. No more counting calories. You don't even have to check to see how many points your dinner with the girls yesterday has set you back. You are now simply eating to feel satisfied.

Step 2
High Satiety Recipes

To further help you focus on the foods that are great for you and that will assist you with this program, I have provided, with the assistance of a professional chef, a two-week long, high-satiety menu that you can use if you want to take even more advantage of the Satiety Index. Here you will find some easy, satisfying recipes for breakfast, lunch, and dinner, plus two snacks. Oatmeal and whole grain cereal are combined in new ways for breakfast on the go. For those mornings, usually weekends, when there's time to slow down and enjoy a leisurely breakfast, try the cottage cheese pancakes or huevos rancheros. Lunch can be a nourishing soup and/or substantial sandwich or perhaps a satisfying grain-based salad. Dinners range from hearty pot pie with a potato topping to a filling lo mein with shrimp and vegetables, to a robust pork tenderloin with baked beans entree. Snacks include pesto-inspired popcorn and granola bars for kids of all ages. Filling. Satisfying. Nourishing. Substantial. Robust. Ample. These words represent the theme of the recipes and all the things you want your food to be. Enjoy and happy weight-loss!

Breakfast

A cup of coffee and a bagel or a doughnut might take the immediate edge off of your early morning hunger, but you really need to eat something hearty and filling to see you through until lunchtime. Oatmeal or whole grain cereal can be microwaved in minutes. Take a scoop of homemade granola or granola bars to work.

For satisfying breakfasts and weekend brunches, huevos rancheros are quickly made with corn tortillas, canned beans, store-bought salsa, and eggs. Cottage cheese pancakes can be made sweet with fruit or savory with onions and herbs.

Apple-Spice Oatmeal

Makes 1 serving

Take the chill out of any morning with a bowl of oatmeal and apple pie flavorings. The recipe can easily be multiplied to serve more people.

INGREDIENTS

½ cup old-fashioned (rolled) oatmeal
Pinch of salt
½ Golden Delicious apple, cored and cut into ½-inch dice
1 tablespoon light brown sugar
1/8 teaspoon apple pie spice or a large pinch each of ground ginger, ground cinnamon, and ground allspice
Milk for serving

DIRECTIONS

1. Combine 1 cup water, oatmeal, and salt together in a microwave-safe medium bowl. Be sure to allow room for the oatmeal to boil up. Microwave on high until the oatmeal is thick, about 3½ minutes. Stir and let stand 1 minute.

2. Combine the apple, brown sugar, and apple pie spice in a small bowl. Sprinkle over the oatmeal. Serve hot, with the milk.

Whole Grain Cereal with
Caramelized Banana

Makes 1 serving

Whole grain cereal may contain anywhere from five to ten different grains—use the one you prefer. But don't confuse it with rolled grain cereal, which is also tasty but similar to oatmeal. This sure beats a cold cereal with a sliced banana any morning.

INGREDIENTS

¼ cup whole grain cereal
Pinch of salt
Canola oil in a pump sprayer or nonstick oil spray
½ banana, peeled and sliced into ¼-inch rounds
2 teaspoons light brown sugar
1 tablespoon seedless raisins
Milk for serving

DIRECTIONS

1. Combine ¾ cup water, cereal, and salt in a 1–quart glass measuring cup or a microwave-safe medium bowl. Be sure to allow room for the cereal to boil up. Cover and microwave on high until the cereal is thick and has absorbed the water, about 5 minutes. Stir and let stand for 2 minutes.

2. Meanwhile, spray the inside of a small nonstick skillet with oil and heat the skillet over medium heat. Add the banana slices and cook for 30 seconds. Turn the banana slices over and sprinkle with the brown sugar. Cook until the sugar melts and the bananas are heated through, about 30 seconds more. Add the raisins.

3. Stir the cereal and transfer it to a bowl. Top with the banana mixture. Serve hot, with the milk.

Good Morning Granola
Makes about 6 cups

Store-bought granolas are often packed with lots of refined sugar and many not-so-good-for-you ingredients. When you make granola, you control what goes into it. Try this recipe then adjust it according to your own tastes, adding more or less of whatever you prefer. Enjoy granola with yogurt, with or without milk for breakfast, or as a between-meal snack.

INGREDIENTS

3 cups old-fashioned (rolled) oats
¾ cup wheat germ
1 cup sliced almonds
½ cup sunflower seeds
½ cup honey
Grated zest and juice of 1 large orange
2 tablespoons canola oil
1 tablespoon ground cinnamon
1 teaspoon vanilla extract
½ teaspoon almond extract
1½ cups seedless raisins or dried cranberries, or a combination

DIRECTIONS

1. Preheat the oven to 300°F.

2. Combine the oats, wheat germ, almonds, and sunflower seeds together in a large bowl. Whisk together the honey, orange zest and juice, oil, cinnamon, and vanilla in another bowl. Pour the honey mixture over the oat mixture and mix well with your hands. Spread in a large-rimmed, foiled-lined baking sheet.

3. Bake, stirring about every 10 minutes, until the mixture is crisp and deep golden brown, about 45 minutes. Cool completely. Stir in the raisins. Transfer to an airtight container and store in a cool, dark place. (The granola can be stored for up to 2 weeks.)

Granola Bars

Makes 12 bars

Too often, granola bars are sugary and taste like candy bars. These easy-to-make bars—a good baking project with kids—are not too sweet. Individually wrap them up for lunchboxes, mid-morning pick-me-ups at work, or snacks on the hiking trail.

INGREDIENTS

2½ cups old-fashioned (rolled) oats
½ cup wheat germ
1 cup coarsely chopped walnuts
1 ½ cups seedless raisins or dried cranberries, or a combination
2 large eggs
⅓ cup honey
3 tablespoons light brown sugar
3 tablespoons unsalted butter, melted, plus more for the baking
    dish
1 teaspoon ground cinnamon
1 teaspoon vanilla extract

DIRECTIONS

1. Preheat the oven to 350°F. Oil a 9 X 13–inch nonstick baking pan. Line the bottom and the short sides of the pan with a 20–inch length of aluminum foil, pleated lengthwise to fit the pan. Oil the foil.

2. Combine the oats, wheat germ, and walnuts on a large rimmed baking sheet. Bake, stirring occasionally, until lightly toasted, 15 to 20 minutes. Transfer to a bowl and stir in the raisins and/or cranberries. Cool slightly. Reduce the oven temperature to 325°F.

3. Whisk the eggs, honey, brown sugar, melted butter, cinnamon, and vanilla together in a bowl. Pour over the oat mixture and mix well. Press evenly into the baking dish.

4. Bake until the edges are beginning to brown, 20 to 25 minutes. Transfer to a wire cake rack and let cool in the pan. Lift up on the foil "handles" and remove the pastry in one piece. Cut into 12 bars.

Cottage Cheese Pancakes
Makes 10 to 12 pancakes

Pancakes made with cottage cheese are lighter than the traditional all-flour version. Here's a sweet version, but if you prefer savory pancakes, omit the sugar and cinnamon and add some sautéed scallions or onions and two tablespoons of chopped herbs such as parsley, cilantro, or mint.

INGREDIENTS

2 cups nonfat cottage cheese
2 large eggs, beaten
¾ cup whole wheat or all-purpose flour
2 tablespoons unsalted butter, melted
1 tablespoon sugar
¼ teaspoon ground cinnamon
Canola oil in a pump sprayer or nonstick cooking spray
Applesauce or maple syrup for serving

DIRECTIONS

1. Stir the cottage cheese, eggs, flour, melted butter, sugar, and cinnamon together in a medium bowl. Let stand for 5 minutes.

2. Heat a large nonstick griddle or skillet over medium heat. Spray with the oil. Using a scant ¼ cup of batter for each pancake, pour the batter into the skillet. Cook until small bubbles appear in the tops of the pancakes and the edges are very lightly browned, about 2 minutes. Carefully turn the pancakes and cook until the other sides are browned, about 2 minutes more. Repeat with the remaining batter.

3. Serve hot with the applesauce.

Huevos Rancheros

Makes 4 servings

Crisp tortillas topped with refried beans, fried eggs, salsa, and cheese make a robust brunch dish. This version uses canned refried beans and store-bought salsa, which also makes the dish easy to put together for a midweek dinner. For quick preparation, heat the beans and salsa in a microwave or in separate saucepans.

INGREDIENTS

4 corn tortillas
Canola oil in a pump sprayer or nonstick cooking oil spray
2 tablespoons olive oil
4 large eggs
Salt and freshly ground black pepper
One 16–ounce can refried beans, heated
1 cup store-bought salsa, warmed
½ cup shredded sharp Cheddar for sprinkling

DIRECTIONS

1. Preheat the oven to 400°F. Spray a large rimmed baking sheet with the oil. Put the tortillas on the baking sheet and spray the tortillas with oil. Bake until crisp, 10 to 12 minutes.

2. Heat the oil in a large skillet over medium-high heat. One at a time, crack the eggs into the skillet and season with salt and pepper. Fry the eggs according to your taste.

3. For each serving, spread each tortilla with about one-fourth of the beans. Put the tortilla on a plate. Top with a fried egg and ¼ cup of the warm salsa. Sprinkle with 2 tablespoons Cheddar and serve hot.

Lunch

Being on the go means that there's often not enough time for a good lunch. Sandwiches can be less than satisfying—some protein slapped between two pieces of processed bread made with refined flours and sugars—and hunger and cravings set in soon after.

To maintain satiety for longer periods of time, think hearty soups, healthy sandwiches on whole grain bread, and nourishing salads made with substantial grains. There's something here for everyone whether lunch is spent at home or at the office. Make the soups on the weekends and pack any leftovers for weekday lunches.

Hearty Bean and Pasta Soup   Makes about 9 servings

Similar to pasta e fagioli, the classic Italian meal in a bowl, this substantial soup is easy to make. If you make it ahead of time, refrigerate and reheat, the soup will become even better.

INGREDIENTS

4 ounces pancetta, prosciutto, or bacon, chopped
2 tablespoons olive oil
1 medium onion, chopped
1 large carrot, cut into ¼-inch dice
1 large celery rib, cut into ¼-inch dice
3 garlic cloves, minced
4 cups canned low-sodium chicken broth
One 28–ounce can diced tomatoes, juices reserved
One 15.5–ounce can red kidney beans, drained and rinsed
One 15.5–ounce can white kidney (cannellini) beans, drained and
    rinsed
½ teaspoon dried rosemary
½ teaspoon dried thyme

1 bay leaf
Salt and freshly ground black pepper
¾ cup whole wheat elbow macaroni
Freshly grated Parmesan cheese for serving

DIRECTIONS

1. Cook the pancetta and oil together in a soup pot over medium
   heat, stirring occasionally, until the pancetta is lightly browned,
   about 10 minutes. Add the onion, carrot, and celery and cover.
   Cook, stirring occasionally, until softened, about 5 minutes. Add
   the garlic and cook until fragrant, about 1 minute.

2. Add the broth, tomatoes and their juices, red and white kidney
   beans, rosemary, thyme, and bay leaf. Season with salt and pepper to taste. Bring to a boil over high heat. Reduce the heat to
   medium-low. Simmer and stir occasionally for about 30 minutes.

3. Meanwhile, bring a large saucepan of salted water to a boil over
   high heat. Add the macaroni and cook according to the package
   directions until al dente. Drain well. Add to the soup and simmer
   for 5 minutes. Remove the bay leaf.

4. Transfer about 2 cups of the soup to a food processor or blender
   and puree until smooth. (If you use a blender, process on low
   speed with the lid ajar.) Stir the puree back into the soup. Ladle
   into bowls and serve hot, passing the Parmesan on the side for
   sprinkling.

White Bean and Sausage Soup   Makes 6 servings

INGREDIENTS

2 tablespoons olive oil

1 medium onion, chopped

2 celery ribs, chopped

2 turkey sausage links (8 ounces total), casings removed

2 garlic cloves, minced

4 cups canned low-sodium chicken broth

Two 15.5–ounce cans white kidney (cannellini) beans, drained and
   rinsed

2 tablespoons chopped fresh parsley, plus more for serving

Salt and freshly ground black pepper

DIRECTIONS

1. Heat the oil in a large saucepan over medium heat. Add the onion
   and celery and cover. Reduce the heat to low and cook, stirring
   occasionally, until the celery softens, about 5 minutes. Move the
   vegetables to one side of the saucepan.

2. Add the sausage to the empty side of the saucepan. Cook, occasionally stirring and breaking up the sausage with the side of a
   spoon, until it loses its raw look, about 6 minutes. Add the garlic
   and cook until fragrant, about 1 minute.

3. Add the broth, beans, and 2 tablespoons of the parsley and season with salt and pepper. Bring to a boil over high heat. Reduce
   the heat to low and simmer until full-flavored, about 30 minutes.
   Mash some of the beans into the soup with a large fork to thicken
   the broth.

4. Ladle into bowls, sprinkle with parsley, and serve hot.

Chicken Salad and Cranberry Wrap   Makes 2 wraps

Sandwiches are too often less-than-satisfying; they're gone in just a few bites and you're still hungry. This ample wrap, however, is filled with enough satisfying flavors to tide you over until dinnertime. Use leftover chicken or purchase a rotisserie chicken from the supermarket. To make an Indian-inspired chicken salad, add ½ teaspoon curry powder.

INGREDIENTS

1½ cups (½-inch) diced cooked chicken
⅓ cup dried cranberries
1 scallion, white and green parts, trimmed and finely chopped
5 tablespoons mayonnaise
2 teaspoons fresh lemon juice
Salt and freshly ground black pepper
Two 10½-inch whole grain tortillas, warmed according to package
    directions
2 large leaves red leaf lettuce

DIRECTIONS

1. Mix the chicken, cranberries, scallion, 3 tablespoons of the mayonnaise, and the lemon juice in a medium bowl. Season with salt and pepper to taste.

2. For each wrap, spread 1 tortilla with 1 tablespoon mayonnaise, leaving a 1–inch border around the edge of tortilla. Cover with a lettuce leave, torn to fit the tortilla. Heap half of the chicken salad in the center of the tortilla. Fold in the sides, then roll up. Cut in half crosswise. Serve at once, or wrap in plastic wrap and refrigerate for up to eight hours.

Roast Beef and Apple Sandwich with
Horseradish Mayonnaise
Makes 1 serving

Just what a sandwich should be—simple, quick and filling. Take it to work for lunch with or without a Thermos of hearty soup. Substitute sliced chicken or turkey for the roast beef.

INGREDIENTS

1 tablespoon mayonnaise
2 teaspoons cream-style prepared horseradish
2 slices whole-grain bread
2 to 3 ounces thinly sliced lean roast beef
½ Granny Smith apple, cored and thinly sliced

DIRECTIONS

1. Combine the mayonnaise and horseradish in a small bowl. Spread over two bread slices.

2. Top 1 slice with half of the sliced apple, the roast beef, and the remaining apple. Cut in half and serve.

Tuna and White Bean Salad
Makes 4 servings

A Tuscan-inspired salad is easy to put together with canned tuna and beans. Enjoy for lunch rolled up in a whole grain wrap or on a bed of fresh greens, or spoon a heaping teaspoon on endive leaves and serve as an appetizer. Substitute basil for the parsley, but add the basil just before serving, as it will discolor if it stands.

INGREDIENTS

Two 15.5–ounce cans white beans (cannellini), drained and rinsed
Two 5 to 6–ounce cans tuna in oil, preferably olive oil, drained and
    flaked

3 ripe plum tomatoes, seeded and cut into ½-inch dice
3 tablespoons minced red onion
3 tablespoons chopped fresh parsley
2 tablespoon red wine vinegar
1 garlic clove, crushed through a garlic press
¼ teaspoon crushed hot red pepper
⅓ cup extra-virgin olive oil
Salt

DIRECTIONS

1. Toss the beans, tuna, tomatoes, red onion, and parsley together in a large bowl.

2. Combine the vinegar, garlic, and hot pepper in a small bowl. Gradually whisk in the oil.

3. Pour the vinaigrette over the bean mixture and toss. Season with the salt. Refrigerate for at least one and up to twelve hours to blend the flavors. Serve chilled or at room temperature.

Niçoise Salad   Makes 4 servings

The perfect summer lunch. Simple to put together and immensely satisfying, especially when served with whole crackers, followed by a bowl of fresh cherries and peaches.

INGREDIENTS

4 ounces green beans, trimmed and cut into ½-inch lengths
10 ounces red-skinned potatoes, scrubbed but unpeeled
½ head romaine lettuce heart, chopped into bite-sized pieces
Two 5 to 6–ounce cans tuna in olive oil, drained and flaked
2 plum tomatoes, seeded and cut into ½-inch dice
⅓ cup pitted and chopped Kalamata olives

3 tablespoons chopped fresh basil or parsley
2 tablespoons red wine vinegar
1 garlic clove, crushed through a garlic press
$1/3$ cup plus 1 tablespoon extra-virgin olive oil
Salt and freshly ground black pepper
1 hard-boiled egg, peeled and chopped

DIRECTIONS

1. Bring a large saucepan of lightly salted water to a boil over high heat. Add the green beans and cook until they are crisp-tender, about 3 minutes. Use a sieve to remove the green beans from the water (keep the water boiling). Rinse the beans under cold running water, drain well, and transfer to a large bowl.

2. Add the potatoes to the saucepan and bring to a boil over high heat. Reduce the heat to medium-low. Cook until the potatoes are tender when pierced with the tip of a sharp knife, about 25 minutes. Drain and transfer to a bowl of cold water. Let stand until cool enough to handle. Drain and cut into ½-inch cubes. Add the potatoes to the bowl with the green beans.

3. Add the lettuce, tuna, tomatoes, olives, and basil and mix together. Whisk the vinegar and garlic in a small bowl. Gradually whisk in the oil. Pour over the salad and toss.

4. Season with salt and pepper to taste. Sprinkle with the chopped egg and serve.

Cold Soba Noodles with
Asian Vegetables

Makes 4 to 6 servings

Served in bowls of hot broth or chilled and tossed with a light Japanese dressing, soba (buckwheat) noodles are filling. Try this salad on a hot summer night when it's too brutal to even turn on the grill. Blanched snow peas, green beans, peas, broccoli florets or other vegetables can be substituted. For a more substantial meal top with cold cooked shrimp or shredded chicken.

INGREDIENTS

12 ounces soba (buckwheat) noodles
3 tablespoons rice vinegar
3 tablespoons soy sauce
3 tablespoons Asian dark sesame oil
2 tablespoons light brown sugar
1 tablespoon peeled and minced fresh ginger
$\frac{1}{8}$ teaspoon crushed hot red pepper
1 cup thawed frozen edamame
$\frac{1}{2}$ red bell pepper, seeds, and ribs discarded, cut into thin strips
$\frac{1}{2}$ seedless cucumber, cut into thin strips
$\frac{1}{2}$ cup chopped fresh cilantro or mint

DIRECTIONS

1. Bring a large pot of salted water to a boil over high heat. Add the soba and cook according to the package directions until barely tender. Drain and rinse well under cold running water to remove any surface starch and discourage the cold noodles from sticking together.

2. Whisk the vinegar, soy sauce, sesame oil, and brown sugar together in a small bowl until the sugar is dissolved. Add the ginger and hot pepper.

3. Toss the noodles, soy sauce vinaigrette, edamame, bell pepper, and cucumber together. Cover and refrigerate until chilled, at least 1 and up to 4 hours. Add the cilantro and serve chilled.

Shrimp Tabbouleh
Makes 6 servings

Tabbouleh, a Middle Eastern bulgur-herb salad, is usually served as an accompaniment to grilled lamb or seafood. But here, shrimp are combined with the bulgur and bright, fragrant herbs for a one-dish lunch or dinner. For a lovely presentation, spoon the tabbouleh into Boston lettuce leaves. Feel free to substitute chicken breast or lean pork for the shrimp.

INGREDIENTS

2 cups boiling water
½ cup bulgur wheat
2 plum tomatoes, seeded and cut into ½-inch dice
2 scallions, white and green parts, trimmed, finely chopped
¼ cup chopped fresh mint
¼ cup chopped fresh parsley
2 tablespoons fresh lemon juice
¼ cup extra-virgin olive oil
1 pound cooked medium shrimp, peeled and deveined

DIRECTIONS

1. Combine the boiling water and bulgur in a heatproof bowl and let stand until the bulgur is tender, about 30 minutes. Drain in a wire sieve.

2. Squeeze the bulgur to remove any excess water. Transfer to a large bowl. Add the tomatoes, scallions, mint, and parsley.

3. Pour the lemon juice into a small bowl and gradually whisk in the olive oil. Pour over the bulgur mixture and toss well. Add the shrimp and toss again. Cover and refrigerate until chilled, about 1 hour. Serve chilled or at room temperature.

Salmon, Orange, and Brown Rice Salad   Makes 4 servings

Roasting is a quick, efficient way to cook salmon fillet. Roast some extra salmon to keep on hand for another meal. Let the salad stand at room temperature for about 30 minutes before serving, because too-cold rice can have an unpleasant texture.

INGREDIENTS

1 pound salmon fillet with skin, pin bones removed
Salt and freshly ground black pepper
2 large seedless oranges
2 cups cooked brown rice (see Note), cooled
2 scallions, white and green parts, finely chopped
½ small red bell pepper, seeds and ribs removed, cut into thin strips
2 tablespoons balsamic vinegar
⅓ cup extra-virgin olive oil, plus more for brushing
2 tablespoons chopped fresh mint, basil, or parsley

DIRECTIONS

1. Preheat the oven to 400°F. Line a rimmed baking sheet with aluminum foil and brush with oil.

2. Brush the salmon with a little olive oil and season with salt and pepper to taste. Place the salmon, skin side down, on the baking sheet. Bake until the salmon is rosy pink when pierced in the thickest part with the tip of a knife, about 15 minutes. Let cool.

3. Grate the zest from ½ orange into a small bowl. Peel the oranges. Cut the oranges crosswise into ½-inch thick rounds, and then bite-sized chunks, discarding any seeds and membrane that get in your way.

4. Toss the brown rice, scallions, red pepper, and orange slices together in a bowl. Flake the salmon into large chunks, discarding the skin. Add to the rice mixture.

5. Add the vinegar to the orange zest in the bowl. Gradually whisk in the oil. Drizzle over the rice mixture and toss again. Season with salt and pepper to taste. Sprinkle with the basil. Serve at cool room temperature.

Cooked Brown Rice:
Bring 3½ cups water, 1½ cups brown rice, and 1 teaspoon salt to a boil in a medium saucepan over medium heat. Reduce the heat to medium-low and cover. Simmer until the rice is tender and has absorbed the water, about 45 minutes. If the water is gone before the rice is tender, add ¼ cup hot water and continue cooking as needed.

Makes about 4½ cups.

Dinner

It may be easier to pick up pizza or Mexican food for dinner on the way home from work, but it sure isn't good for you. With that in mind, here are some easy-to-prepare, healthy recipes that use quality convenience foods and don't take much time to get on the table. They'll feed four people at one sitting, or you can enjoy leftovers for lunch the next day.

Whole Wheat Linguine with
Shrimp and Feta   Makes 4 to 6 servings

Baked shrimp topped with crumbled feta, a classic Greek combination, is nestled on a bed of whole wheat linguine for a filling main course.

INGREDIENTS

1 pound whole wheat linguine
4 tablespoons olive oil
1 pound medium shrimp, peeled and deveined
2 garlic cloves, minced
1½ pints grape tomatoes, halved lengthwise
3 scallions, white and green parts, thinly sliced
¾ cup chopped pitted Kalamata olives
¼ cup chopped fresh basil or 2 tablespoons chopped fresh
    oregano
¾ cup (3 ounces) crumbled feta
Salt and freshly ground black pepper

DIRECTIONS

1. Bring a large pot of salted water to a boil over high heat. Add the linguine and cook according to the package directions until al dente.

2. Meanwhile, heat 2 tablespoons of the oil in a large skillet over medium-high heat. Add the shrimp and cook, stirring often, until they turn opaque, about 2 minutes. Transfer to a bowl.

3. Add the remaining 2 tablespoons of oil to the skillet and heat. Add the garlic and cook just until softened, about 30 seconds. Add the tomatoes, scallions, and olives and cook until the tomatoes are heated through and give off their juices, about 3 minutes. Stir in the shrimp and basil.

4. Drain the linguine, reserving ½ cup of the cooking water. Return to the pot and add the tomato mixture and add the feta. Toss, adding enough of the reserved cooking water to moisten the pasta. Season with salt and pepper to taste. Serve hot.

Whole Wheat Macaroni and Cheese   Makes 8 servings

The choice is usually between mac 'n cheese from a box (which bears no resemblance to the real thing at all) or a complicated recipe that requires several pots and hours. Here's a quick version that can be on the table in an hour or so.

INGREDIENTS

1 pound whole wheat elbow macaroni or ziti
1 pint cottage cheese
2 large eggs
¼ cup milk
2 teaspoons Dijon mustard
½ teaspoon salt
¼ teaspoon freshly ground black pepper
3 cups (12 ounces) shredded sharp Cheddar
1 cup fresh whole-grain breadcrumbs (make in a blender or food processor)
2 tablespoons unsalted butter, melted, plus more for the baking dish

DIRECTIONS

1. Preheat the oven to 350°F. Butter a 9 X 13–inch baking dish.

2. Bring a large pot of salted water to a boil. Add the macaroni and cook according to the package directions until tender. Drain well.

3. Combine the cottage cheese, eggs, milk, mustard, salt, and pepper in a food processor or blender and process until smooth. Transfer to a large bowl. Add the macaroni and cheese and mix well. Spread in the baking dish.

4. Toss the breadcrumbs with the butter. Sprinkle over the macaroni. Bake until the sauce is bubbling and the crumbs are golden brown, about 25 minutes. Serve hot.

Baked Potatoes with Chili

Makes 4 servings

INGREDIENTS

Four 7–ounce baking potatoes, scrubbed

2 tablespoons olive oil

1 medium onion, chopped

½ medium green bell pepper, seeds and ribs discarded, cut into
 ¼-inch dice

2 garlic cloves, minced

1 jalapeño, seeded and minced (optional)

2 tablespoons chili powder

1 pound ground sirloin

One 8–ounce can tomato sauce

½ teaspoon salt

Shredded Cheddar for serving

DIRECTIONS

1. Preheat the oven to 400°F. Pierce each potato a few times with the tip of a sharp knife. Put the potatoes directly on the oven rack and bake until tender when pierced with a knife, about 45 minutes.

2. Meanwhile, heat the oil in a large saucepan over medium heat. Add the onion and bell pepper and cook, stirring occasionally, until softened, about 5 minutes. Add the garlic and jalapeño, if using, and cook until fragrant, about 1 minute. Add the chili powder and stir for 15 seconds.

3. Add ground sirloin and cook, stirring often and breaking up the meat with the side of a spoon, until it loses its raw look, about 10 minutes. Stir in tomato sauce and salt and bring to a boil. Reduce the heat to medium-low and simmer until the chili thickens, about 20 minutes.

4. For each serving, put a potato in a bowl and make a long slit down the center. Press from opposing ends to make the potato burst open. Top with the chili, sprinkle with cheese, and serve hot.

Mediterranean Cod-Potato Cakes   Makes 4 servings

Fishcakes are substantial and a good way to use up leftover cod or any other white fish, such as flounder or halibut. If you don't have leftover cod, season two six-ounce cod fillets with salt and pepper. Heat 1 tablespoon olive oil in a large nonstick skillet over medium-high heat. Add the cod and cook, turning once, until the cod is lightly browned and it looks opaque when flaked in the thickest part with the tip of a knife, about 8 minutes.

INGREDIENTS

Two 7–ounce baking potatoes, peeled and cut into 2–inch chunks
1 tablespoon olive oil, plus more in a pump-spray bottle
1 small onion, finely chopped
2 garlic cloves, minced
2 tablespoons chopped fresh cilantro, basil, or parsley
3 large eggs
2 cups flaked cooked cod fillets
½ teaspoon salt
¼ teaspoon freshly ground black pepper
1½ cups whole wheat breadcrumbs, made in a blender or food
   processor from day-old crusty bread
Lemon wedges for serving

DIRECTIONS

1. Preheat the oven to 400°F. Lightly oil a rimmed baking sheet.

2. Put the potatoes in a large saucepan and add enough salted water to cover by 1 inch. Cover the pot and bring to a boil over high heat.

Reduce the heat to medium-low and remove the lid. Cook until the potatoes are tender when pierced with the tip of a knife, about 25 minutes. Drain well. Transfer to a bowl and mash with a potato rice or a hand-held electric mixer. Cool slightly.

3. Meanwhile, heat 1 tablespoon of the oil in a large skillet over medium heat. Add the onion and cook, stirring occasionally, until translucent, about 4 minutes. Stir in the garlic and cook until the garlic is fragrant, about 2 minutes. Add to the mashed potatoes, along with the cilantro, and stir. Beat 1 egg and stir into the mashed potato mixture. Add the cod, salt, and pepper and mix well.

4. Shape equal amounts of the cod mixture into 8 cakes. Beat the remaining 2 eggs in a shallow dish. Spread the breadcrumbs in another dish. Coat each cake in the eggs, then the breadcrumbs. Place the cakes on the baking sheet.

5. Spray the cod cakes with olive oil. Bake until crispy and heated through, about 20 minutes. Serve hot, with the lemon wedges.

Salmon with Crunchy Potato Crust   Makes 4 servings

The crunchy crust wrapped around tender salmon is made with crushed potato chips! Put whole potato chips in a plastic bag, seal, and crush with a rolling pin or flat skillet.

INGREDIENTS

Four 5– to 6–ounce salmon fillets
Salt and freshly ground black pepper
1 tablespoon mayonnaise
Grated zest of ½ lemon
²/₃ cup coarsely crushed potato chips
Lemon wedges for serving

DIRECTIONS

1. Preheat the oven to 400°F. Lightly oil a rimmed baking sheet.

2. Season the salmon lightly with salt and pepper to taste. Mix the mayonnaise and lemon zest together. Spread a thin layer of the mayonnaise mixture over the meaty side of each salmon fillet. Put the potato chips in a plate. One at a time, mayonnaise-side down, place a salmon fillet in the potato chips and press gently to coat the meaty side with chips. Arrange the fillets, skin-side down, on the baking sheet.

3. Bake until salmon is rosy pink when pierced in the thickest part, 8 to 10 minutes. Serve hot, with the lemon wedges.

Brown Rice Shrimp Paella

Makes 4 servings

INGREDIENTS

2 tablespoons olive oil

1 medium onion, finely chopped

½ red bell pepper, seeds and ribs discarded, finely chopped

2 garlic cloves, minced

2 teaspoons sweet paprika

½ teaspoon crumbled saffron

¼ teaspoon crushed hot red pepper

1½ cups long-grain brown rice

5 cups canned low-sodium chicken broth

1 cup dry white wine

½ teaspoon salt

1 pound large shrimp, peeled and deveined (or 3 dice chicken breasts if you prefer)

One 10–ounce package thawed frozen artichoke hearts

½ cup thawed frozen baby peas

Chopped fresh parsley for serving

Lemon wedges for serving

DIRECTIONS

1. Heat the oil in large, deep skillet over medium heat. Add the onion and red bell pepper and cook, stirring often, until softened, about 5 minutes. Stir in the garlic and cook until it is fragrant, about 1 minute. Stir in the paprika, saffron, and hot pepper.

2. Add the rice and stir well. Add the broth, wine, and salt. The liquid should be about ½ inch above the rice; add water as needed. Stir and bring to a boil over high heat.

3. Reduce the heat to medium-low and cover. Simmer until the rice is almost tender (there will still be liquid in the skillet), about 35 minutes.

3. Uncover the skillet and place the shrimp on the rice (do not stir), and top with the artichokes hearts and peas. Cover again and cook until the shrimp are opaque and the brown rice is tender, about 10 minutes. Remove from the heat and let stand, covered, for 5 minutes.

4. Sprinkle with the parsley. Serve hot, directly from the skillet, with the lemon wedges.

Grilled Chicken Breast with
Grapefruit-Avocado Salad
Makes 4 servings

Whether cooked outdoors over coals or indoors in a grill pan, always make extra chicken breasts to keep on hand for salads and sandwiches.

Grapefruit-Avocado Salad
INGREDIENTS

2 large grapefruit, cut into sections (see Note)
1 ripe avocado, pitted, peeled, and cut into ½-inch dice
1 tablespoon chopped fresh tarragon
Grated zest of 1 lime
1 tablespoon fresh lime juice
1 tablespoon extra-virgin olive oil
Salt and freshly ground black pepper

Four 6–ounce boneless and skinless chicken breast halves

2 teaspoons ground cumin
1 teaspoon salt
½ teaspoon freshly ground black pepper

DIRECTIONS

1. To make the salad, gently stir the grapefruit sections, avocado, tarragon, lime zest and juice, and oil together in a medium bowl. Season with salt and pepper to taste. Cover and let stand at room temperature while grilling the chicken.

2. Build a medium-hot fire in an outdoor grill.

3. Lightly pound the chicken breast halves with a meat mallet or rolling pin until they are evenly thick. Mix the cumin, salt, and pepper together and sprinkle all over the chicken.

4. Lightly oil the grill grate. Place the chicken on the grill and cover. Grill until sear marks appear on the underside, about 4 minutes. Turn and grill just until the chicken springs back when pressed, about 3 minutes more.

5. For each serving, place a chicken breast on a dinner plate. Using a slotted spoon, divide the salad evenly among the plates. Serve immediately.

Note: To cut grapefruit into segments, trim the top and bottom off the grapefruit so it stands on the work counter. Using a serrated knife, cut off the thick peel where it meets the flesh so you end up with a skinless sphere. Working over a medium bowl to catch the juices, hold the fruit in one hand, cut between the thin membranes to release the segments, and let the segments fall into the bowl. Squeeze the juices from the membranes into the bowl.

Chicken Pot Pie with Garlicky
Potato Topping

Makes 4 servings

No-crust pot pie is easy to put together. Mashed potatoes, freshly cooked or leftover, seal in the chicken and vegetables.

INGREDIENTS

1½ pounds baking potatoes, such as Russet or Burbank, peeled and cut into 2–inch chunks

12 garlic cloves, peeled

1 tablespoon vegetable oil

1 pound boneless and skinless chicken thighs, cut into bite-sized pieces

1 medium onion, chopped

2 medium carrots, cut into ¼-inch dice

2 medium celery ribs, cut into ¼-inch dice

4 tablespoons unsalted butter, plus more for the baking dish

1¾ cups canned low-sodium chicken broth

3 tablespoons whole wheat flour

1 cup thawed frozen corn kernels

2 tablespoons chopped fresh parsley

Salt and freshly ground black pepper

¼ cup milk, heated

DIRECTIONS

1. Preheat the oven to 350°F. Butter an 8–inch square baking dish.

2. Put the potatoes and garlic in a large saucepan and add enough salted water to cover by 1 inch. Cover with a lid and bring to a boil over high heat. Reduce the heat to medium-low. Simmer, uncovered, until the potatoes are tender when pierced with the tip of a knife, about 25 minutes.

2. Meanwhile, heat the oil in a large skillet over medium-high heat. Add the chicken thighs and cook, stirring occasionally, until the chicken is lightly browned, about 6 minutes. Add the onions, carrots, celery, and 2 tablespoons of the butter. Cover and reduce the heat to medium. Cook, stirring occasionally, until softened, about 5 minutes.

3. Whisk the broth and flour together to dissolve the flour. Pour into the skillet and add the corn. Bring to a boil. Reduce the heat to medium-low and simmer until the sauce thickens slightly, about 5 minutes. Season with salt and pepper to taste. Pour into the baking dish.

4. Drain the potatoes and garlic and transfer to a bowl. Using a potato masher or hand-held electric mixer, mash the potato mixture with the milk and remaining 2 tablespoons butter. Season with salt and pepper to taste. Dollop the mashed potatoes over the chicken mixture. Put the dish on a baking sheet.

5. Bake until the sauce is bubbling and the topping is tipped with brown, about 20 minutes. Serve hot.

Chinatown Fried Rice

Makes 4 servings

The secret to making topnotch fried rice is to use cold, leftover rice. Hot rice sticks together; each grain should be coated with soy sauce. Add leftover diced chicken or shrimp.

INGREDIENTS

2 tablespoons canola oil
3 large eggs
Pinch of salt
1 cup diced smoked ham
2 scallions, white and green parts, finely chopped
½ cup thawed frozen peas
3 cups cold cooked brown rice (see page 131)
3 cups fresh bean sprouts
3 tablespoons soy sauce

DIRECTIONS

1. Heat a very large nonstick skillet or wok over high heat. Add the oil and swirl to coat the inside of the skillet. Beat the eggs and salt together in a small bowl and set aside.

2. Add the ham and stir-fry until lightly browned, about 1 minute. Add the scallions and peas and stir-fry for 30 seconds. Add the rice and bean sprouts and stir-fry until the rice is beginning to heat through, about 2 minutes.

3. Move the rice mixture to one side of the skillet. Add the beaten eggs to the empty side of the skillet and stir until they are scrambled, about 20 seconds. Add the soy sauce to the rice mixture, then mix together with the scrambled eggs. Serve hot.

Shrimp and Vegetable Lo Mein   Makes 4 servings

The ingredients list of any stir-fry can look long, but once the ingredients are prepared, the cooking goes very quickly. Substitute or add vegetables of your choosing.

INGREDIENTS

8 ounces whole wheat spaghetti
½ cup canned low-sodium chicken broth
4 tablespoons soy sauce
2 teaspoons sugar
¼ teaspoon crushed hot red pepper
4 tablespoons canola oil
12 ounces medium shrimp, peeled and deveined
1 tablespoon peeled and minced fresh ginger
2 garlic cloves, minced
½ medium red bell pepper, seeds and ribs discarded, cut into thin
    strips
1 medium zucchini, cut into thin 2–inch long strips
1 medium carrot, cut into thin 2–inch long strips
2 scallions, white and green parts, trimmed and cut into 1–inch
    lengths
2 teaspoons Asian dark sesame oil

DIRECTIONS

1. Bring a large pot of salted water to a boil over high heat. Add the spaghetti and cook according to the package directions until tender. Drain and rinse under cold running water. Toss with 1 tablespoon of the canola oil.

2. Mix the broth, soy sauce, sugar, and hot pepper together in a small bowl; set aside.

3. Heat a large wok or skillet over high heat. Add 1 tablespoon of the canola oil, swirl to coat the inside of the wok, and heat until the oil is very hot. Add the shrimp and stir-fry until they turn opaque, about 2 minutes. Transfer to a platter.

4. Add the remaining 2 tablespoons of canola oil to the wok and heat. Add the ginger and garlic and stir-fry until fragrant, about 10 seconds. Add the red bell pepper, zucchini, and carrot, and stir-fry until softened, about 1 minute. Add the spaghetti and stir-fry until the spaghetti is heated, about 1 minute. Stir the soy sauce mixture and add to the wok, along with the shrimp and scallions. Stir-fry until the scallions are wilted, about 1 minute. Transfer to the platter, drizzle with the sesame oil, and serve hot.

Fish Tacos with Apple Slaw
Makes 4 servings

Meaty cod is the best fish to use when making these tacos. Fish tacos are often made with fried fish, but broiled cod is just as good—and there's no mess. Broiling the fish works better than grilling; the fish doesn't fall into the fire. If you do grill the fish, use a perforated grilling sheet.

Apple Slaw
INGREDIENTS

One 1–pound bag cole slaw mix
1 Granny Smith apple, peeled, cored, and shredded on the large holes of a box grater
2 scallions, white and green parts, trimmed and chopped
½ cup mayonnaise
2 tablespoons fresh lime juice
2 tablespoons chopped fresh cilantro (optional)
Salt and freshly ground black pepper

Fish

¼ cup olive oil
2 tablespoons fresh lime juice
1 tablespoon chili powder
¼ teaspoon salt
1 pound cod fillets
16 corn tortillas, heated

DIRECTIONS

1. To make the slaw, combine the cole slaw mix, shredded apple, scallions, mayonnaise, lime juice, and cilantro, if using. Season with salt and pepper to taste. Let stand at room temperature for 1 hour to blend the flavors.

2. Combine the oil, lime juice, chili powder, and salt in a large zippered plastic bag. Add the cod and turn to coat in the marinade. Refrigerate for 30 minutes.

3. Position a broiler rack 6 inches from the source of heat and preheat the broiler. Lightly oil a broiler pan.

4. Remove the cod from the marinade. Arrange on the broiler pan. Broil the cod until lightly browned, about 3 minutes. Turn (don't worry if the cod breaks) and continue broiling until the cod is opaque when pierced in the thickest part with the tip of a knife, about 3 minutes more. Transfer to a bowl and break into large chunks.

5. Serve the cod, tortillas, and cole slaw. For each taco, stack 2 tortillas and fill with the fish and cole slaw.

Spice-Rubbed Pork Tenderloin with Baked Beans

An updated spin on pork and beans, but this version is made with spiced and roasted pork tenderloin and can beans.

INGREDIENTS

One 1–pound boneless pork tenderloin, silver skin trimmed
2 teaspoons sweet paprika, preferably smoked paprika, such as
    Pimentón de La Vera
1 teaspoon ground cumin
1 teaspoon dried oregano
1 teaspoon salt
¼ ground hot red (cayenne) pepper
One 28–ounce can baked beans, heated

DIRECTIONS

1. Build a medium-hot fire in an outdoor grill.

2. Fold the thin tip of the tenderloin over and tie it with kitchen string so the tenderloin is equally thick from end to end. Mix the paprika, cumin, oregano, salt, and pepper together in a small bowl. Rub all over the pork.

3. Lightly oil the grill grate. Place the pork on the grill and cover. Grill, turning occasionally, until a meat thermometer inserted in the thickest part of the pork reads 145°F, about 20 minutes. Transfer the pork to a cutting board and let stand 5 minutes.

4. Slice the pork across the grain, with the knife held at a slight diagonal, into ½-inch thick pieces, discarding the string. Serve the sliced pork with the baked beans.

Grilled Flank Steak with
Mango-Tomato Salsa

Makes 4 servings

INGREDIENTS

¼ cup olive oil
2 tablespoons Worcestershire sauce
2 garlic cloves, minced
½ teaspoon freshly ground black pepper
1½ pounds flank steak

Mango-Tomato Salsa
INGREDIENTS

1 ripe mango, pitted, peeled, and diced
2 ripe plum tomatoes, seeded and diced
1 scallion, white and green parts, finely chopped
2 tablespoons chopped fresh cilantro or mint
2 tablespoons fresh lemon juice
1 jalapeño, seeded and minced
Pinch of salt

DIRECTIONS

1. To marinate the steak, whisk the oil, Worcestershire sauce, garlic, and pepper together in a bowl. Pour into a zippered plastic bag. Score the steak in a diamond pattern with a sharp knife, making the slashes about ⅛–inch deep and 2 inches apart. Add the steak and close the bag. Refrigerate, turning occasionally, for at least 1 and up to 8 hours.

2. To make the salsa, combine the mango, tomatoes, scallion, cilantro, lemon juice, jalapeño, and salt in a medium bowl. Mix and let stand at room temperature for 1 to 2 hours to blend the flavors.

3. Build a hot fire in an outdoor grill. Lightly oil the grill grate. Remove the steak from the marinade. Grill, turning once, until the steak is well-browned on both sides, about 6 minutes for medium-rare meat. (Flank steak is too thin to test for doneness with an instant-read thermometer, and flank steak dries out if it is cooked more than medium-rare.)

4. Transfer the steak to a cutting board and let stand for 5 minutes. Carve across the grain, with the knife held at a slight diagonal, into thin slices. Serve hot, with the salsa passed on the side.

The Two Week High Satiety Menu

There are two secrets to maintaining good eating habits: Plan ahead and stock the pantry. If you have vegetables and fruits in the crisper; shrimp, chicken, and lean meats in the freezer; and grains, canned beans, and whole pasta in the cabinet, cooking recipes in this book will be easy. With some menu planning and a well-stocked pantry, you'll be less likely to eat processed foods that aren't good for you.

Below are some suggested menus to help with meal planning. We've all heard that we should eat more vegetables and fruits — at least five a day. To reach that goal, have a salad as a main course or as a side dish. A green salad can be put together in minutes!

Keep apples, pears, berries, melons, kiwi, and other fruits on hand. Cut up fruit and keep it in a bowl in the fridge. Enjoy with a few spoonfuls of nonfat plain yogurt for a between-meal snack.

Week 1

Monday

BREAKFAST Good Morning Granola with Nonfat Plain Yogurt

LUNCH Hearty Bean and Pasta Soup • Crusty Whole Wheat Roll • Orange

DINNER Grilled Chicken Breast with Grapefruit-Avocado Salad • Cooked Brown Rice

Tuesday

BREAKFAST Apple-Spice Oatmeal

LUNCH Roast Beef and Apple Sandwich with Horseradish Mayonnaise

DINNER Chinatown Fried Rice • Orange Wedges

Wednesday

BREAKFAST Whole Grain Cereal with Caramelized Banana

LUNCH Cold Soba Noodles with Asian Vegetables

DINNER Spiced Rub Pork Tenderloin with Baked Beans • Apple Slaw (ingredients on page 146)

Thursday

BREAKFAST Granola Bar • Fruit Salad

LUNCH Salmon, Orange, and Brown Rice Salad • Mixed Berries

DINNER Baked Potatoes with Chili • Sauteed Spinach

Friday

BREAKFAST	Apple-Spice Oatmeal • Grapefruit Juice
LUNCH	Niçoise Salad • Fresh Fruit Salad
DINNER	Chicken Pot Pie with Garlicky Potato Topping

Saturday

BREAKFAST	Cottage Cheese Pancakes • Mixed Berries
LUNCH	White Bean and Sausage Soup • Granola Bar
DINNER	Brown Rice Shrimp Paella

Sunday

BREAKFAST	Huevos Rancheros • Cut-up Cantaloupe
LUNCH	Cold Soba Noodles with Asian Vegetables • Orange Wedges
DINNER	Salmon with Potato Crust • Steamed Broccoli

Week 2

Monday

BREAKFAST	Granola Bar • Citrus Fruit Salad
LUNCH	Chicken Salad and Cranberry Wrap • Orange
DINNER	Mediterranean Cod-Potato Cakes • Steamed Asparagus

Tuesday

BREAKFAST   Apple-Spice Oatmeal

LUNCH   Shrimp Tabbouleh • Grapefruit-Avocado Salad
(Ingredients on page 140)

DINNER   Grilled Flank Steak with Mango-Tomato Salsa •
Chinatown Fried Rice

Wednesday

BREAKFAST   Good Morning Granola with Nonfat Yogurt

LUNCH   Roast Beef and Apple Sandwich with Horseradish
Mayo

DINNER   Grilled Chicken Breast • Cooked Brown Rice

Thursday

BREAKFAST   Whole Grain Cereal with Caramelized Banana

LUNCH   Tuna and White Bean Salad • Strawberries

DINNER   Whole Wheat Linguine with Shrimp and Feta •
Side Salad

Friday

BREAKFAST   Granola Bar • ½ Grapefruit

LUNCH   Cold Soba Noodles with Asian Vegetables

DINNER   Salmon with Crunchy Potato Crust

Saturday

BREAKFAST   Huevos Rancheros

LUNCH   Hearty Bean and Pasta Soup • Niçoise Salad

DINNER   Shrimp and Vegetable Lo Mein

Sunday

BREAKFAST   Cottage Cheese Pancakes

LUNCH   Shrimp Tabbouleh • Sliced Tomatoes

DINNER   Spice-Rubbed Pork Tenderloin with Baked Beans •
Apple Slaw (ingredients on page 146)

Chapter 11

LEVEL 3
THE SENSA
FASTERCIZE SYSTEM

As we have mentioned before, people gain weight when they take in more calories over time than they expend and they lose weight when they expend more calories over time than they take in. One of the keynote methods to expend more calories is through exercise.

One of the major themes of the Sensa Weight-Loss Program is minimal, gradual changes to your lifestyle. Any drastic changes will disrupt your "comfort zone" and the result will be that you will return to your normal routines in a very short period of time. There is no surprise in knowing that your daily exercise is also influenced by your comfort zone as well. Nothing causes a more dramatic disruption in your lifestyle than going from zero exercise to a very intense, lengthy exercise routine on a daily basis. This not only dramatically disrupts your routine but also inflicts a high level of pain into your life in various forms. I know a number of people who wanted to succeed so much that they went from being totally sedentary to trying to run five miles the first day of their new routine. Nothing could set you up for failure more than this.

Human energy (calorie) expenditure (EE) is the amount of energy expended or calories burned by the body and can be broken down into three basic types. The first is you Basal Metabolic Rate (BMR) that I explained in a previous chapter. This is the amount of energy that your body uses up on a daily basis if you remained completely sedentary all day—without one movement. If you are in a sedentary occupation such as office work, then your BMR could make up approximately 60% of your daily EE. Your BMR is largely determined by your Body Mass Index as explained before. The more you weigh, the more energy your body expends on a daily basis just by remaining in a listless position.

The second type of EE that your body uses is the thermic effect of food (TEF). TEF is the increase in EE associated with the digestion, absorption, and storage of food and accounts for approximately 10% to15% of total daily EE.

The third type of EE that your body uses is activity thermogenesis (AT). This type is composed of energy that we expend from exercise activity thermogenesis (EAT) and non-exercise activity thermogenesis (NEAT). EAT relates to designated, specific exercise routines that you take part in to burn calories, control weight, and attain better health. NEAT relates to the normal course of daily activities that you take part in such as walking, climbing stairs, getting up from a chair, doing dishes, etc. NEAT is composed of an enormous variety of activities that are centered on occupation, leisure activities, and fidgeting. Yes, I said fidgeting.

Have you ever had a friend that couldn't seem to keep still? He or she talks on their cell phone and they have to pace back and forth. They can't sit in a chair for five minutes before they have to get up. They speak fast, move their hands around and walk fast. These are the fidgeters of the world and are blessed with being able to expend more energy and burn more calories on a daily basis than you.

If BMR makes up 60% of EE and TEF contributes 10% to 15% of EE, then that leaves us with 25% to 30% being contributed by AT—exercise and non-exercise related activities that we perform on a daily basis. But the interesting part is that even for active exercisers, NEAT contributes by far the majority percentage of energy burn. Go back and read the beginning of this chapter again because I want you to understand the ramifications of this. **What I am saying is that you have a better chance of burning more calories on a daily basis with changes to your non-exercise related activities (NEAT) then with your routine-specific, exercise activites.** In an interesting study conducted at the Mayo Clinic, 20 sedentary individuals were studied to determine how different activity levels contributed to different levels of weight.[28] In the study, one group of participants (five men and five women) had an average BMI of 23 (lean), while the other 10 men and women had an average BMI of 33 (mildly obese). What researchers found was very interesting:

- The obese group sat for 164 minutes longer each day than the lean group.
- The lean people were upright for 153 minutes longer than the obese people.

- The lean group burned an average of 350 extra calories each day (36 lbs a year) by walking and standing more throughout the day.

Though neither group did any structured exercise, the lean group burned extra calories just by moving around more without sweating.

Does this mean that exercise is not important? Absolutely not. But by making some conscious, gradual, easy changes in your daily activities, you can dramatically increase your ability to burn calories and lose weight.

All of this being said, the Sensa Fastercize System is composed of two steps. The first step involves gradually incorporating more NEAT (non-exercise) activites into your daily routine; the second step introduces you to a customizable, formal exercise program to increase your EAT calorie burn. Both steps follow the premise of minimizing the impact to your lifestyle.

Step 1—NEAT Activities

NEAT activities involve gradually incorporating simple, non-strenuous energy expending routines into your daily life. As shown above, these activities can go a long way to maximizing and maintaining your weight loss over time. The following list of 25 NEAT activities can be totally customizable to your lifestyle. You should, in no way, view it as a list that has to be completed every day. Everyone's lifestyle and work environment is different. Even if you just incorporate one of the activities below into your routine, it will have a significant impact over time.

1. SIT UP STRAIGHT IN CHAIRS—Believe it or not, sitting up straight expends more calories than slouching. Be conscious of this whenever you sit.

2. STAND UP AND WALK AROUND WHEN YOU TALK ON THE PHONE—Even if you have a corded phone, you can stand up and pace a little back and forth.

3. CARRY GROCERIES IN THE STORE—Obviously if you have a large amount of groceries to buy, this wouldn't be feasible, but if you just need a few items, grab a hand basket to use. You would be surprised how many people use a wheeled cart to buy one or two items.

4. PARK YOUR CAR IN THE FARTHEST PARKING SPACE AND WALK—How many times have you driven around over and over again to gain a space that is one or two closer to your destination? Think of how much easier it would be mentally to not be concerned about getting the closest space. In addition, you will be burning so much more energy to boot.

5. FOLLOW #4—But walk around the parking lot or block once before going into your destination.

6. DO THE FOLLOWING IF YOU ARE SITTING FOR A PERIOD OF TIME:

- Shift in your seat
- Stretch

- Squeeze your hands together
- Contract your abs

All of these make lengthy sitting more tolerable and you burn energy at the same time.

7. GET UP TO CHANGE THE CHANNEL MANUALLY—This is probably very difficult to do if you are a man because the remote control has become such a huge extension of your anatomy, but try it a few times a week. You may be surprised how easy it seems.

8. BRING IN ONE BAG OF GROCERIES AT A TIME—Instead of carrying two, limit it to one. You will make a few more trips, but each trip will be a little easier.

9. WALK AROUND THE HOUSE—You probably feel like you do this already but how many times have you just sat around the house most of the day. Get up and move around periodically.

10. WASH YOUR CAR BY HAND—Although it may not be as good for the environment as a car wash, doing this once or twice a month definitely can burn some energy. If you're concerned about the environment, use a manual car wash where you do all the work.

11. WALK FASTER—Pick up your pace whenever you do walk.

12. WALK UP AND DOWN THE STAIRS IN YOUR HOUSE FOR NO REASON—This is a great way to burn calories and you may catch your children doing something that they shouldn't be doing as a bonus.

13. PLAY WITH YOUR CHILDREN LONGER—We all know how much energy this expends. If you typically spend 15 minutes a day playing with them, extend it to 30 minutes or an hour. Your kids will love it and your body will as well.

14. PUT ON SOME MUSIC AND DANCE—This is a fun way to burn plenty of calories.

15. WALK AROUND THE MALL WINDOW SHOPPING—Walking becomes a fun activity when you are distracted by all the great products in the shop windows not to mention people watching. If the mall is close by, walk to it instead of driving.

16. PREPARE MEALS AT HOME—Taking the time to chop, stir and serve is not only a good way to eat healthier, but all of the prep work helps burn calories as well.

17. GET OFF A STOP EARLY AND WALK—If you take public transportation, get off a stop early and walk the distance. If you get a ride from a friend, get out a block or two before your destination and walk.

18. WALK TO SEE SOMEONE INSTEAD OF EMAILING THEM—Today, email has replaced snail mail but it has also decreased human contact with each other. In some cases, you can get so much more accomplished by just walking over to someone and dealing with the issue directly. Try it a few times a day. You may make some new friends in the process.

19. GO FOR A WALK ON YOUR LUNCH BREAK—Leave some extra time and take a brief 15 minute walk before or after lunch.

20. WALK TO A RESTROOM ON ANOTHER FLOOR—If you work in an office building, walk to another floor to use the restroom. In fact, you can walk up a flight of stairs when you get to work and take the elevator from there. Do the same when you leave work.

21. TAKE A FAMILY WALK AFTER DINNER—Make this a regular activity to get the family together and help to digest your food at the same time.

22. GET UP AND WALK AROUND THE OFFICE—If you work in an office, you can tend to get so ingrained in your work that you remain sedentary all day. Get up a few times during the day and walk around. This may also help you to get to know more of what's going on in the company.

23. BIKE—If you don't have a bike, buy one and use it for short errands instead of the car or just take a leisurely ride once in a while.

24. STRETCH—Stretch when you wake up and before you go to bed. In fact, make it a regular habit to stretch throughout the day.

25. GET UP EVERY CHANCE YOU GET—Today we sit for far greater periods than we have in the past. Make it a habit to get up periodically, stretch and walk around. Your body will love you for it.

These are just a few of the activities that you can perform. Have some fun. Get creative and design your own personal list of NEAT activities below that would be more attuned to your individual lifestyle. Make a real effort to complete them every day.

Personal NEAT Activities

1. _____

2. _____

3. _____

4. _____

5. _____

6. _____

7. _____

8. _____

9. _____

10. _____

The purpose of step 1 (NEAT) of the Sensa Fastercize System is to make you more cognizant of simple activities that you can incorporate into your daily routine that when accomplished over time can pay incredible dividends as far as weight loss and control is concerned. Again, begin to incorporate one, some, or all of these into your daily life at your own pace. Don't feel that you have to do them all at once or even do them all. Mix them up. Do some one day and some the next. Have some fun. Take real pleasure in doing them. There are no rules here. The goal is to burn more calories in a simple, non-threatening way.

Step 2—EAT Activities

Exercise means a set of planned, structured and repetitive bodily movements in order to improve or maintain physical fitness. As an element of health, exercise involves both strength training of the muscles and cardiovascular fitness, with stretching activities for flexibility. Losing weight is about so much more than eating less. Every study shows that adding a fitness or exercise component to a weight-loss plan is important to the success of any program and to your overall well-being. Exercise not only helps us keep up our physical health, but it just plain feels good. Exercise releases endorphins, hormones in the brain that induce euphoria, or what some athletes refer to as a natural high. A fitness regime builds strong muscles and bones, imparts higher energy levels, and delivers better sleep patterns, all of which improve life in endless ways.

But exercise also has challenging aspects to it. It can dramatically change your lifestyle. You have to set out a certain time to do this on a regular basis. If you have lived a sedentary lifestyle, it dramatically takes you out of your comfort zone. It can also inflict pain as you begin to use muscles in different ways

If you look at any exercise routine, it is composed of three factors—frequency, intensity, and time. In today's society, one of the most limiting factors to performing any exercise routine on a regular basis is time. I was very aware of this when I developed the exercise plan.

Exercise Plan

The following exercises do not require any special equipment and can be done in less than 20 minutes a day. Simply pick one exercise from each of the 4 exercise groups and mix-and-match to create a combination that's right for you. Start by doing only 2 sets of 10 repetitions and then increase your intensity by either adding a third set or increasing the repetitions to 12 or 15. While these exercises were developed with an expert trainer, I always recommend consulting your physician before beginning any exercise program.

To increase intensity or add more to your workouts, use the Bonus Exercises and include a 5th exercise to your training sessions. For better results, do this four to five times a week. Recovery days are very important, so remember to take a couple of days off each week and let your body rest.

Warming Up

Before you start each exercise routine, it is important to warm up your muscles. This will prepare your body for the strength training and lessen any risk of injury. I suggest taking 5 minutes before each work out to go for a quick walk. Whether it is moving around the house, walking up the stairs a couple of times, or maybe even cleaning the kitchen—your body will ease into the routine and maximize the results.

Cooling Down

It is equally important to give yourself a stretching period after each work out. Here are a few easy stretches to complete each set:

Stretching Menu

PRONE STRETCH FOR YOUR ABDOMINAL MUSCLES
Lie face down on a mat or padded surface. Place both hands flat on floor directly next to your shoulders. Keep your legs on the floor and your toes pointed. Slowly extend your arms until your arms reach a full-extended position. Hold for 10 seconds, release and repeat 2 more times.

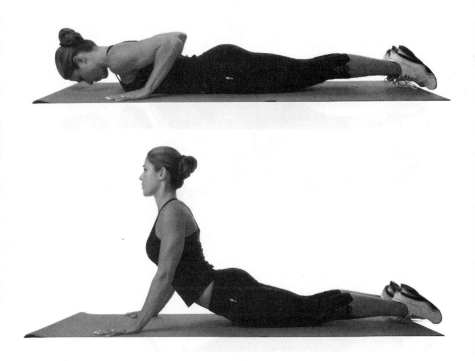

SUPINE STRETCH FOR YOUR BACK

Lie flat on your back on a mat or padded surface. Keeping your legs together, slowly raise your knees and bring them close to your chest. Reach both arms behind your legs and grip tight. As you pull your arms closer you will feel a deeper stretch through your back. Perform this stretch very slowly. Hold for 10 seconds, release and repeat 2 more times.

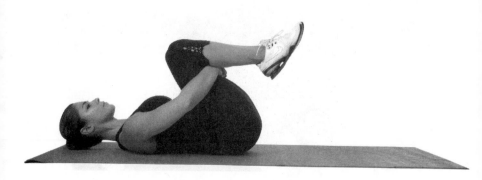

KNEELING SLIDE BACK STRETCH FOR YOUR
ARMS AND SHOULDERS

Kneel down on a mat or padded surface and keep your buttocks close to your heels. Start with your hands on your knees and slowly begin to walk your hands forward until your arms become fully extended. Keep your head down and your neck aligned with your spine. Hold the stretch for 5 seconds and return to start position. Repeat 3 more times.

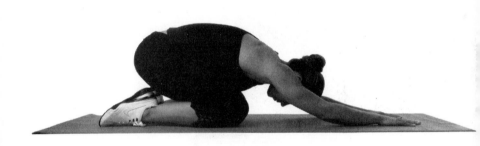

STANDING WALL STRETCH FOR YOUR LEGS AND CALVES

Stand about 15 inches from the wall. Bend your knees and place the back of your forearms on the wall as you slowly lean forward. Move one foot back and place the entire foot on the floor keeping that same leg extended. Hold for 10 seconds, return to start position and switch legs. Alternate the leg stretch 2 times on each side.

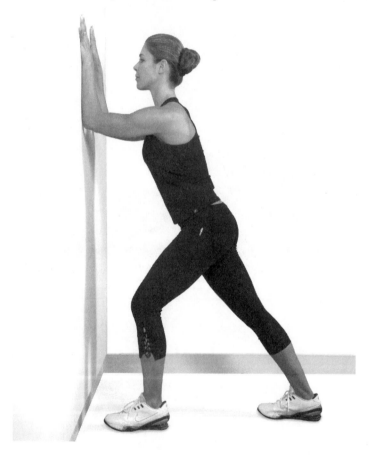

STANDING STRETCH FOR YOUR QUADRICEPS

Stand next to a sturdy chair or a wall. Grip the chair with one hand. Keeping your left knee slightly bent, lift your right foot up off the floor and bend the right knee back. Reach back with the right hand and grasp your right foot. Pull gently and be careful not to over stretch the right knee. Hold for 5 seconds, release, and switch to the left side for the same stretch. Repeat this stretch 2 more times on each side.

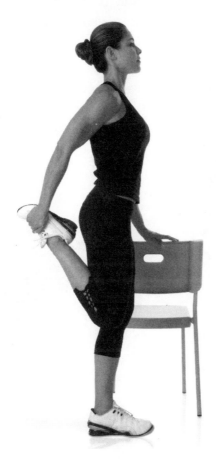

Exercise Group 1
Primary focus on Legs

CHAIR ASSISTED SQUATS

This type of squat uses a chair to help your body learn the motion of a proper squat. Start with your feet shoulder-width apart and stand directly in front of a chair. Lift your arms forward and keep your knees slightly bent. Without arching your back, move your arms forward, begin to squat slowly until your body is about 1 to 3 inches from the chair and then return to the starting position.

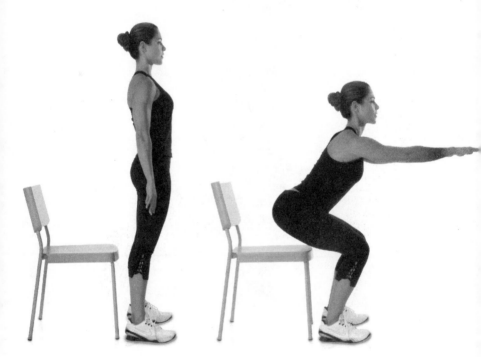

WALL SQUATS

Place your entire back on a sturdy and smooth wall or door. Take a step forward and begin the exercise by lowering your body down to a squat position keeping your knees behind your toes during the lower phase of the exercise. Hold the down phase for 2 seconds before pushing your body back up to the starting position.

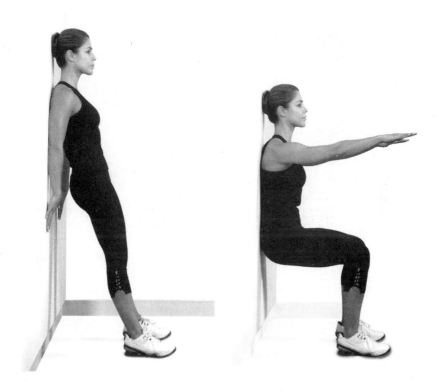

PLIE SQUATS

Start with your feet wider than your hips and your toes turned out to the sides. (Slightly wider than a "V" position). Place your hands together and reach your arms forward. Slowly lower your body down until the back of your legs reach as close to a 90–degree angle as possible. Return to the start position slowly.

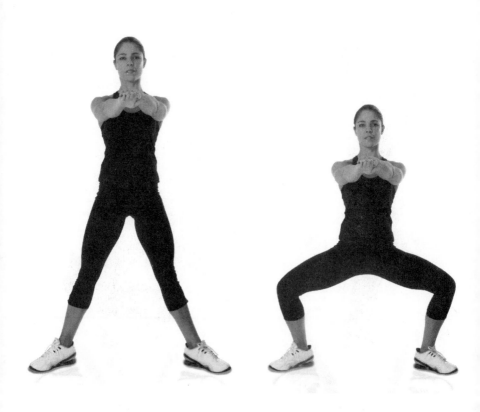

SQUATS

Start with your feet facing forward, slightly wider than your hips. Without arching your back, begin to squat slowly keeping your knees aligned forward and behind your toes. Simply hold your arms down and make sure your heels do not lift up from the ground as you squat down.

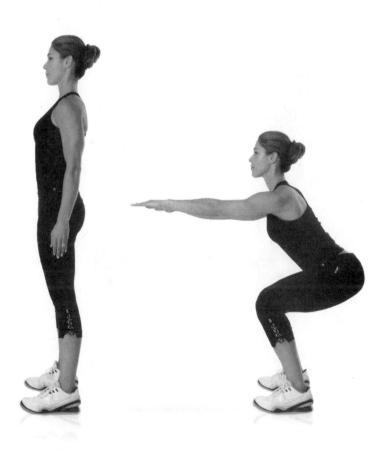

Exercise Group 2
Primary focus on Arms

STANDING BICEP CURLS (NARROW)
Start with your feet shoulder-width apart and begin by moving your hands upward until just past a 90–degree angle. Lower your hand again to the starting position. This exercise will be done by counting "4" on your way up and "4" on your way up. Add resistance by squeezing your hands into a fist position.

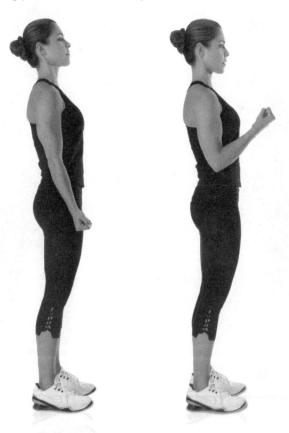

STANDING BICEP CURLS (WIDE)

Start with your feet shoulder-width apart. Lower your elbows down to your waist level and move your hands out to a wide position. Begin by moving your hands upward until just past a 90–degree angle. Lower your hand again to the starting position. This exercise will be done by counting "4" on your way up and "4" on your way down. Add resistance by squeezing your hands into a fist position.

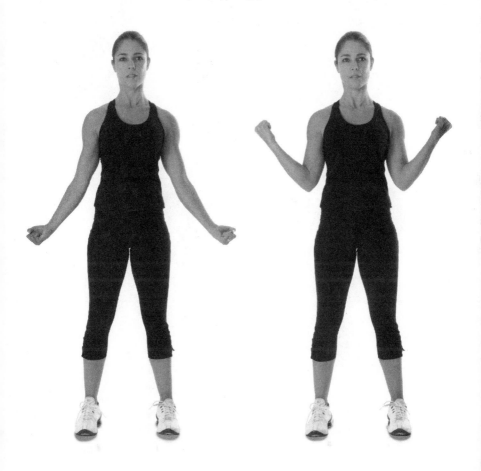

TRICEP KICKBACKS

Start with your feet shoulder width-apart and your knees bent. Lean your upper body slightly forward and lift your elbows back. Begin by extending your forearm back until your arm is almost straight and return to the start position.

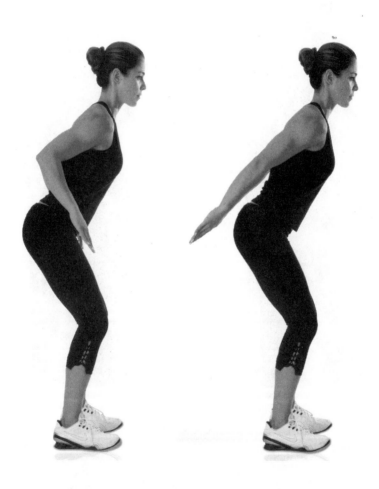

OVERHEAD TRICEP EXTENSIONS

Start with your feet facing forward, slightly wider than your hips. Keep your back straight and elevate your arms directly above your head. Cross your hands together and lower your forearms behind you without moving your elbows out of position. Return your arms to the top position and repeat the same motion.

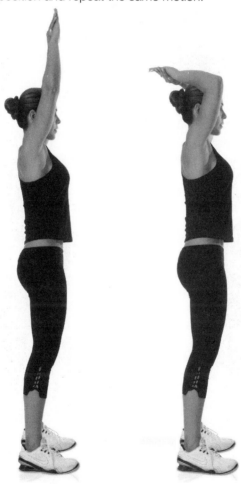

Exercise Group 3
Primary focus on Shoulders

LATERAL RAISE

Slowly separate your feet until they are shoulder-width apart and place your arms down along the side of your body. Elevate both arms out without locking your elbows until they reach shoulder level. Bring arms down to start position and repeat. Add resistance by creating a fist position with your hands.

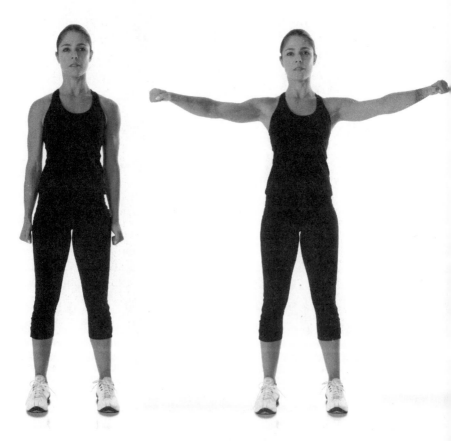

SHOULDER PRESS

Slowly separate your feet until they are shoulder-width apart. Bring your arms up to your shoulders. Begin by elevating both arms above your head as if you were pushing the ceiling upward. Reach up to full extension without locking your elbows. Return to start position and repeat.

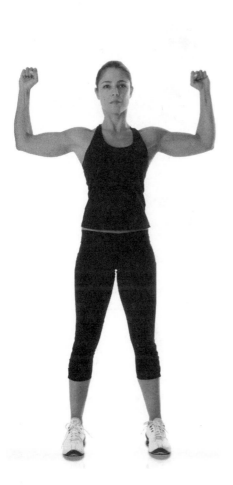
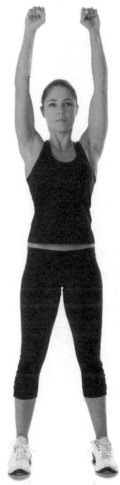

FRONT RAISE

Start with your feet shoulder width-apart and your knees bent. Bring both arms directly in front of you. Begin by raising your arms straight-forward until they reach your shoulder level. Bring arms down to starting position and repeat. Add resistance by creating a fist position with your hands.

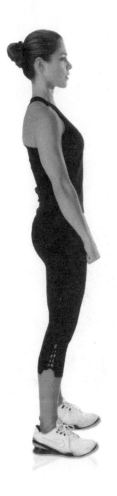 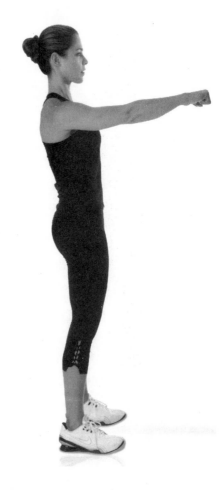

REAL DELTOID PUSH-BACKS

Start with your feet facing forward, slightly wider than your hips. Open the palm of your hands and extend your arms behind you. Begin by pushing your arms back without locking your elbows. Keep a short motion without leaning your body forward. Bring your arms back to the starting position and repeat.

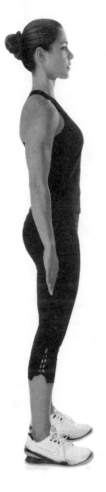
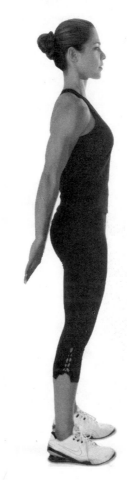

Exercise Group 4
Primary focus on Abs

CRUNCHES

Lie on a mat or padded surface. Bend your knees to a 90 degree angle and keep your heels on the floor. Reach your hands back and gently touch your fingers to the back of your head with your elbows out. Without pulling on your neck, crunch upward and slowly return to the start position. This exercise will be done by counting "2" on your way up and "2" on your way down. Take a 30 second break between each set of ten repetitions.

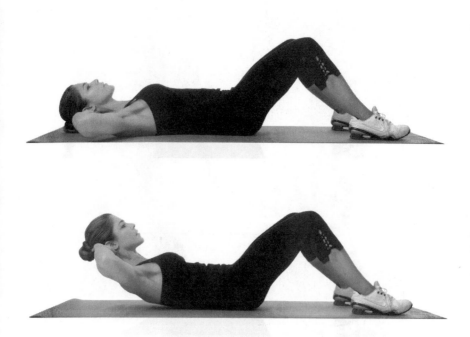

REVERSE CRUNCHES

Lie on a mat or padded surface with your arms by your side and palm of the hands down. Walk your heels up to your gluteus as close as you can. Once your heels are close to your buttocks, lift them up about 5 inches from the ground. This is your starting position. Now bring your knees toward your chest as you keep your knees bent. This exercise will be done by counting "4" on your way up and "4" on your way down. Take a 30 second break between each set of ten repetitions.

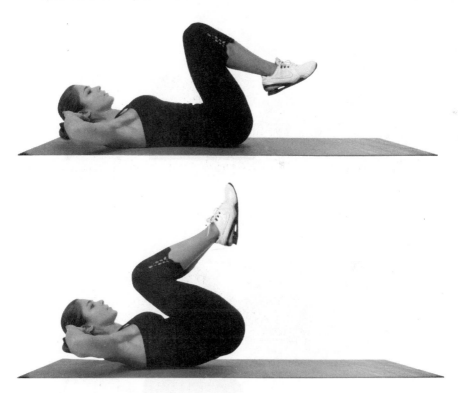

BICYCLE CRUNCHES

Lie flat on your back on a mat or padded surface. Place your hands behind your head without pulling on your neck. Slightly bend your knees and raise your heels from the ground. Keeping your abs tight and your chin up, begin moving your right elbow to your left knee and rotate your left elbow to your right knee slowly. You will "pedal" for 15 seconds before resting for 30 seconds.

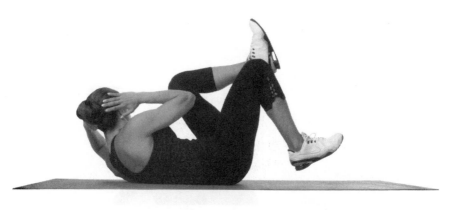

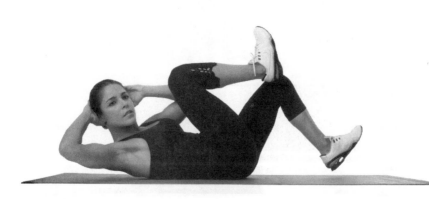

SEATED RUSSIAN TWISTS

Sit on a mat or padded surface with your knees bent and feet
together. Reach your hands forward, facing your knees. Now slowly
rotate your torso from side to side without elevating your feet or gluteus from the ground. Repeat 10 rotations to each side, 3 times.

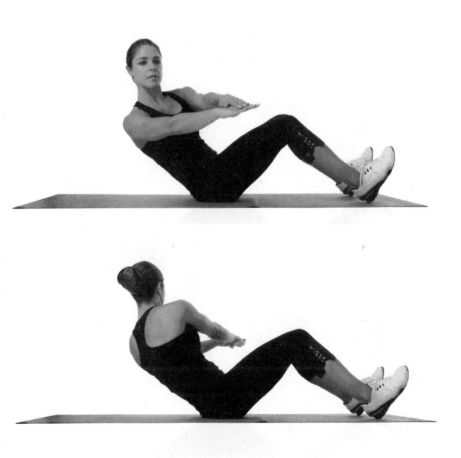

Exercise Group 5—Bonus Exercises
You can intensify your workout by adding one or more of the following exercises to your routine.

POWER SQUAT KNEE LIFT
Start with your feet wider than your shoulders and reach both of your arms forward. Lower your upper body down without allowing your knees to go over your toes. On your way back up, elevate the right knee. Repeat the same exercise and alternate by elevating the left knee.

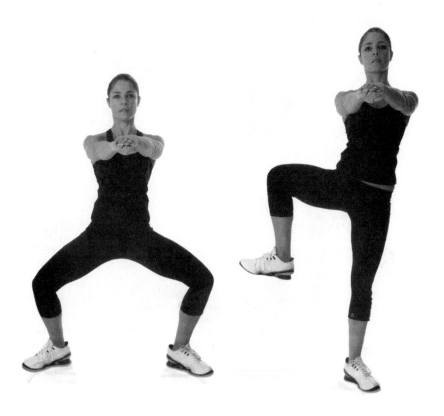

ASSISTED LUNGES

Find a sturdy chair for balance. Stand on the back side of the chair with one hand on your hip and the other resting on the back of the chair. Starting at a split lunge position, lower your body down and elevate your body back up. Perform the lunge 8 times on each leg. Please note that to avoid injury, make sure that your front knee does not bend beyond a 90–degree angle and does not move forward past your toes.

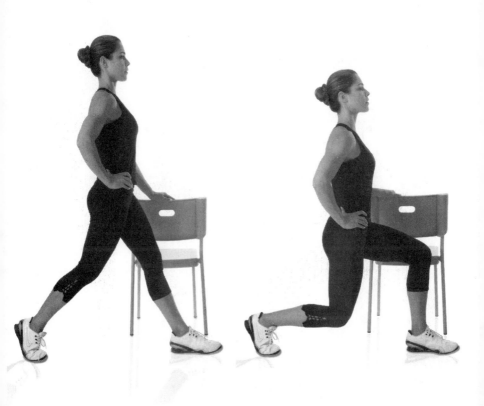

STEP-UPS!

For this exercise you will need to find a step. This can be a curb, the first step of your staircase, or an exercise step platform. Start by facing the step with both feet on the ground. Place your right foot up and lift to elevate your left knee up.

Step down to the floor with your left foot. Alternate your right foot and repeat the exercise with the left foot on the step. Do this 20 times. (10 times on each foot). Take a 30 second break and repeat this 2 more times for a total of 3 Sets of 20 alternating knee lifts. To add resistance, extend the opposite arm as you step up.

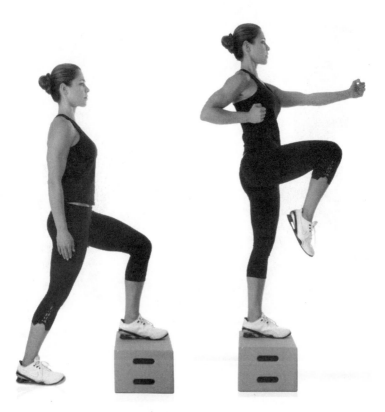

STANDING INCLINE PUSH-UPS

Start by standing close to wall and placing your hands shoulder width apart on the wall slightly lower than your shoulders. Take 3 to 4 steps back as you keep your hands on the wall. You will be on a slight incline position. Make sure your feet are secure and will not slip back. Now allow your arms to lower your body toward the wall until your elbows are close to the side of your body. Now push yourself back to the beginning position. This exercise will be done by counting "4" on your way down and "4" on your way up. Perform 3 sets of 10 repetitions and only take a 30 second break between each set.

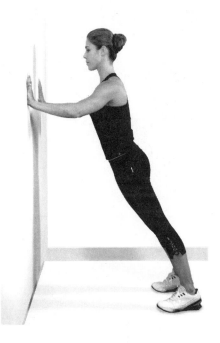
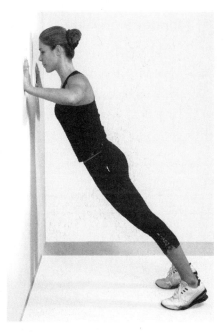

As you start to incorporate these exercises into your life, remember that this is customizable and designed for convenience. I know how difficult it is to carve out 20–30 minutes in my day between work, kids, and making time for my spouse. However, we all deserve "me time." Making these minor changes in your life will have major impact on your weight and hopefully self-esteem. Exercise releases endorphins—endorphins make us happy—and isn't that the ultimate goal?

Sample Workout

Monday workout

- Warm Up (Walk for 5 minutes)
- Wall Squats (from Exercise Group 1): 2 sets of 10 repetitions
- Tricep Kickbacks (from Exercise Group 2): 2 sets of 10 repetitions
- Lateral Raises (from Exercise Group 3): 2 sets of 10 repetitions
- Oblique Crunches (from Exercise Group 4): 2 sets of 10 repetitions
- Cool Down (stretching)

Chapter 12

PUTTING IT ALL TOGETHER

Thank you for spending the past few hours, days, or weeks with me while I have attempted to make a dream of mine come true—developing a simple, effective, clinically-proven program to help people like you who are struggling with weight loss. I hope I have provided you with a roadmap to begin your own journey toward achieving your own personal weight goals.

While I am aware that this new concept of using your sense of smell and taste to combat weight loss may have seemed strange before you read this book, I hope you have a better understanding of how these two senses play a significant role in many aspects of our lives, including our weight. Bestselling author, Dr. Robert Schuller has stated this simple premise—"inch by inch, it's a cinch. Yard by yard it's hard." The Sensa Weight-Loss Program is an "inch by inch" program. I do not promise you instant results or dramatic results in a short period of time. **What I do believe is that Sensa will be the easiest, simplest and most effective way for you to achieve and maintain your weight-loss goal.**

You've learned a lot. Now how do you put it all together? Remember, The Sensa Weight-Loss Program is composed of three levels and the timing of when you begin each level is completely up to you. While it is certainly OK to start all three levels at the same time, it is not recommended. The success of the program is based on easing yourself into each level gradually. The following is meant to present an example of how to accomplish this.

Level 1—The Sensa Tastant System

Always start with the Sensa Tastant System—Level I, described in Chapter 8. **Remember that the Tastants work differently for everyone.** Some people start to see results immediately. For others, the weight loss may take longer. The key is to stick with it. There is no disruption to your lifestyle other than remembering to sprinkle the Tastants on everything that you eat. This will be the most difficult part. Use some reminders to help you with this that were suggested in that chapter as well. As you start to see weight loss, you will become more cognizant of what you are eating and you may start to notice new eating habits emerging during this time: you may start snacking less, you may not be able to eat as much at each meal and you may crave healthier foods. As your clothes start to fit a little better and your friends compliment your slimmer physique, you may feel the motivation to get out and start moving.

This is a great point to start Level 2. While you are feeling better about yourself and seeing real results, you'll find yourself excited to start the next part of your journey. For some people, that may be a loss of five pounds. For others, it may be ten pounds. Some people may not get excited before they lose fifteen or twenty pounds. Excitement equals motivation. Motivation equals action—the action to advance to the next level.

Level 2—The Sensa Satiety System— Step 1: High Satiety Foods

As your motivation kicks in, it is the perfect time to start substituting higher satiety foods for some of the lower satiety foods that you are currently eating. For example, substitute multi-grain, whole wheat bread when you have a sandwich, have an orange for a snack instead of a banana, eat jelly beans instead of a candy bar. All of these are simple, minor changes that you can begin to incorporate into your daily lifestyle. At this point, you are still using the Sensa Tastants but you are sprinkling them on some new foods. You are more cognizant of the foods that you are eating. You see additional success on the program by losing even more weight. Maybe you have to go out and buy a few new articles of clothing because your old ones don't stay on your body as well or they appear too loose (What a great problem this is!)

Level 2—The Sensa Satiety System— Step 2: High Satiety Recipes

While you have been making some smaller substitutions, now is a great time to start cooking high satiety meals. Start out with a few new breakfast items—then incorporate some new meals at lunch and dinner. Go as slowly or as quickly as you like. You may be eating out at restaurants and you are making better menu choices that will keep you satisfied longer. Eventually, you may try to prepare all two weeks worth of Sensa Satiety menu items. However, don't forget to continue using the Sensa Tastants. Your friends are asking you about your new lifestyle. They are noticing that you are ordering differently in restaurants than you did before and might be motivated by your new outlook. Along the way, you are continuing to lose weight and feeling great about your progress. Now is the time to begin Level 3. Remember there is no right or wrong time to do this—it's completely up to you. It is more about "feeling" right about it than feeling pressured to start when you aren't ready.

Level 3—The Sensa Fastercise Program— Step 1: NEAT Activities

Start incorporating several of the NEAT activities outlined in Chapter 11. You start parking your car in the furthest parking spot. You stand up when you speak on the phone. You sit up straight in chairs. You spend more time in the mall just walking around and window shopping. You walk up a flight of stairs before you get on an elevator. When confronted with an escalator, you choose the stairs instead. Your husband or wife comes home one day and finds you dancing by yourself. You have more energy. You go to the doctor for a checkup and your blood pressure is down. All the while, you continue to use the Sensa Tastants on everything you eat. You're feeling so well that you are ready to start a formal exercise program to burn even more calories. It's time to incorporate EAT exercise activities into your daily routine as explained in Level 3 of the program.

Level 3—The Sensa Fastercise Program— Step 2: EAT Activities

Start by incorporating Sensa exercises into your lifestyle just a couple of days a week. Take it slow. As the workouts become easier and you find more time in your schedule, you can build up to a five-day-a-week program. You are in the best shape you have been in a long time and you're loving life. Your friends are so impressed that they want to do the program with you. You have finally arrived at your ideal weight and you feel better than you ever have.

Congratulations! You have completed the Sensa Weight-Loss Program. What's next? Possibly, enter a marathon or climb Mount Everest. The world is at your feet. Welcome to your new life—your Sensa life!

About the Author

Alan R. Hirsch, M.D., F.A.C.P., a Neurologist and Psychiatrist specializing in the treatment of smell and taste loss, is the Neurological Director of the Smell & Taste Treatment and Research Foundation in Chicago. He is a Faculty Member in the Department of Medicine at Mercy Hospital and Medical Center, and Assistant Professor in the Departments of Neurology and Psychiatry at Rush University Medical Center. Dr. Hirsch is certi- 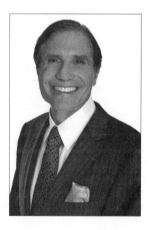 fied by the American Board of Neurology and Psychiatry in Neurology, Psychiatry, Pain Medicine, Geriatric Psychiatry, and Addiction Psychiatry.

Dr. Hirsch conducts in depth studies of the chemosensory system and its relation to all aspects of life. Some examples include studies observing the effects of aromas on behavior, emotions, mood, and interactions between individuals.

An inventor and investigative researcher in the areas of smell and taste, Dr. Hirsch frequently lectures across the country and has extensively published many of his studies' findings. He has served as an expert on smell and taste for *CNN, Good Morning America, Dateline, The Oprah Winfrey Show, CBS Early Show,* and *Extra.*

Additionally, Dr. Hirsch is a member of numerous professional organizations, including the American Academy of Neurology, American College of Physicians, the American Medical Association, the Association of Chemoreception Sciences, the National Association for Holistic Aromatherapy, and Editorial Committee of *The International Journal of Essential Oil Therapeutics.* He has served on the Editorial Advisory Board of *The International Journal of Aromatherapy,* Associate Editor of *Neurology Healthcare USA,* the Advisory Board of the National Academy of Sports Medicine, the Medical Advisory Board of Chronic Fatigue Syndrome Society of Illinois, and on the Editorial Advisory Board of the Professional Journal of Sports Fitness/CPT News.

Dr. Hirsch received both his B.A. and M.D. degrees from the University of Michigan in Ann Arbor and completed his residencies in both Neurology and Psychiatry at Rush University Medical Center in Chicago.

Also a prolific author, Dr. Hirsch has written several books, *Dr. Hirsch's Guide To Scentsational Weight Loss, Scentsational Sex, What Flavor Is Your Personality?, Life's A Smelling Success, What*

Your Doctor May Not Tell You About Sinusitis, and *What's Your Food Sign?*

Dr. Hirsch's twenty-plus years of research regarding the impact of smell and taste on weight loss led him to develop the patent-pending technology used today in the *Sensa Weight-Loss System.* He conducted one of the largest studies of a non-prescription weight-loss system to test the effectiveness of *Sensa* as a means of weight-loss.

Resources

Sensa Weight-Loss System
(www.trysensa.com)

Visit the Sensa website for more detailed information on how to use and purchase the Sensa Tastants. Once you have purchased Sensa, you can become part of the Sensa community and read what others have to say about their experience with Sensa. There are active message boards, logs and journals to download, and expert advice from the Sensa team to further assist you on your weight-loss journey.

The Smell & Taste Treatment and Research
Foundation (www.smellandtaste.org)

Founded by Dr. Alan Hirsch, the Smell & Taste Treatment and Research Foundation specializes in the evaluation, diagnosis and treatment of smell and taste-related disorders. In addition, the staff's research extends to the effects of odors and flavors on human emotion, mood, behavior and disease states. Dr. Hirsch has performed several studies on the effects of smell and taste on weight loss, sleep, consumer preferences and sexual habits, among many other topics.

The Centers for Disease Control (www.cdc.gov/healthweight/assessing/bmi)

Body Mass Index (BMI) is a number calculated from a person's weight and height. BMI provides a reliable indicator of body fatness for most people and is used to screen for weight categories that may lead to health problems. The above link will lead you directly to the CDC's web page that will allow you to calculate your BMI.

Hilton Publishing (www.hiltonpub.com)

Since 1996, Hilton Publishing has been providing patient-education material that is written for the layperson. You can visit the Hilton Publishing website for information on various illnesses that may affect you and your family. The website also contains an "Ask the Doctor" section that provides quick answers from leading doctors and surgeons.

References

Chapter 2

1. Greenemeier, Larry, "Vaccine makers await critical swine flu samples; Swine flu won't be in seasonal flu vaccines." *Scientific American*, www.scientificamerican.com (posted 4/29/09).
2. Robbins, Liz and Grady, Denise, "Outbreak in Mexico may be smaller than feared." *The New York Times*, http://www.nytimes.com/2009/05/03/health/03flucnd.html (posted 5/2/09)
3. National Center for Health Statistics. Chartbook on Trends in the Health of Americans. Health, United States, 2006. Hyattsville, MD: Public Health Service. 2006. Statistics Related to Overweight and Obesity http://www.win.niddk.nih.gov/STATISTICS/
4. Centers for Disease Control and Prevention, and http://www.wrongdiagnosis.com/o/obesity/stats.htm.

5. Barness LA, Opitz JM, Gilbert-Barness E (December 2007). "Obesity: genetic, molecular, and environmental aspects". *Am. J. Med. Genet. A 143A* (24):3016-34.doi:10.1002/ajmg.a.32035. PMID

6. http:www.who.int/dietphysicalactivity/publications/facts/obesity/en/

7. http:www.who.int/dietphysicalactivity/publications/facts/obesity/en/

8. Centers for Disease Control and Prevention. U.S. Obesity Trends, Trends by State, 1985-2008. http://www.cdc.gov/obesity/data/trends.html (accessed May 2009).

9. http:www.healthnetwork.com.au/weight-loss/obesity.asp

10. Pawlik-Kienlen, Laurie (July 2007). "Mental Health Effects of Obesity: *The Psychological Consequences of Being Overweight Vs. Underweight.*" http://psychology.suite101.com/article.cfm/mental_health_effects_of_obesity (accessed May 2009)

Chapter 3

11. Sawer, Patrick. "Fat people blamed for global warming." http://www.telegraph.co.uk/news/1973230/Fat-people-blamed-for-global-warming.html (posted May 17, 2008).

12. Farah, Hodan and Buzby, Jean. "U.S. Food Consumption Up 16 Percent Since 1970." http://www.ers.usda.gov/AmberWaves/November05/Findings/USFoodConsumption.htm

13. http://www.mayoclinic.com/health/calories/WT00011

14. U.S. Department of Health and Human Services. Fact sheet (January 2007) http://www.surgeongeneral.gov/topics/obesity/calltoaction/fact_glance.htm (accessed May 2009).

15. For Preschoolers Even Play Tends to be Sedentary. Based on a study published in *Child Development*, Jan/Feb issue. http://www.bio-medicine.org/medicine-news-1/For-Preschoolers--Even-Play-Tends-to-Be-

Sedentary-35997-1/ (posted February 2009).

16. U.S. Department of Health and Human Services. Fact sheet (January 2007). http://www.surgeongeneral.gov/topics/obesity/calltoaction/fact_glance.htm (accessed May 2009).

17. *The Economist* (February 2009). The American Association for the Advancement of Science, "What's Cooking?" http://www.economist.com/science/displayStory.cfm?story_id=13139619

18. Bray, George A., Nielsen, Samara Joy, and Popkin, Barry M., "Consumption of high- fructose corn syrup in beverages may play a role in the epidemic of obesity" (American Journal of Clinical Nutrition, Vol. 79, No. 4, 537-540, April 2004). http://www.ajcn.org/cgi/content/full/79/4/537 (accessed May 2009)

19. Ibid.

20. Ibid.

21. Lean, Geoffrey, Pollution can make you fat, study claims. *The Independent* online, http://www.independent.co.uk/life-style/health-and-wellbeing/health-news/pollution-can-make-you-fat-study-claims-921696.html (posted September 2008).

22. Musante, Kenneth, Prescription drug sales rate hits 47-year low. http://money.cnn.com/2008/03/12/news/prescription_sales/index.htm (posted March 2008).

23. Goodman, Brian M., Study Suggests 10 New Obesity Causes: America's Weight Problem Not Due To Gluttony And Sloth Alone, Researchers Say, http://www.cbsnews.com/stories/2006/06/27/health/webmd/main1757772.shtml (posted June 2006).

24. BBC News, Obesity linked to lack of sleep, http://news.bbc.co.uk/2/hi/health/4073897.stm (posted December 2004).

Chapter 6

25. Macbeth, Helen M., *Food Preferences & Taste* (Berghahn Books, 1997, 978-1571819581), pg. 42.
26. Rolls, E.T. and Rolls, J.H. (1997) Olfactory Sensory-Specific Satiety in Humans. *Physiology and Behavior* 61(3):pp. 461-473. Oxford e-prints, http://eprints.ouls.ox.ac.uk/archive/00000937/ (accessed May 2009).

Chapter 8

27. Dorland's Medical Dictionary. Saunders, 2007.

Chapter 11

28. Levine, James A., et. al. Interindividual Variation in Posture Allocation: Possible Role in Human Obesity. *Science Magaine*, January 28, 2005 (Vol. 307, No. 5709, pp. 584)

Index

Acknowledgments

This book would not have been possible without the unselfish, generous, and kind efforts of some very special people. I wish to thank the thousands of people who participated in the studies that culminated in the knowledge needed to write this book. I thank current and past staff members for their hard work on studies and research. Special kudos to Denise Fahey for her Herculean efforts and without whose devotion, this book would never have come to fruition and Michele Soto for her selfless efforts in fulfilling the unreasonable demands of this project. My special thanks and gratitude go to Hilton M. Hudson, II, M.D., Rockelle Henderson, and Harriet Bell for their contributions in perfecting this manuscript. Noteworthy also are the contributions of Kimberly Tobman, Bob Johnson, Matt Lueders, and especially, Don Ressler, whose support, encouragement, and friendship were unwavering. Most of all, I thank my wife Debra and our children Marissa, Jack, Camryn, and Noah, for their encouragement and understanding in allowing me to take the time from our lives together to complete this project.

Special Reader Offer!

Get 15% off on your first purchase of the Sensa Weight-Loss System Tastants.

Go to **www.sensabookoffer.com** and follow instructions.

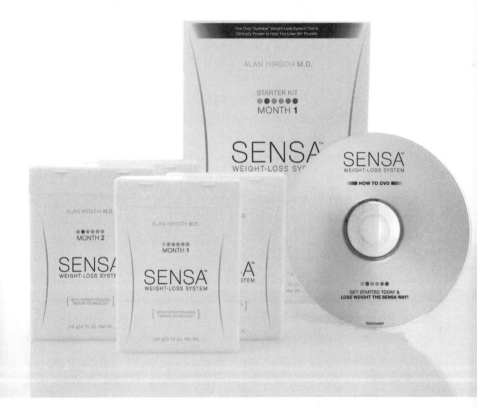

NOTES

NOTES